HOMOEOPATHY IN THE LIGHT IF MODERN SCIENCE

HOMOEOPATHY
IN THE LIGHT OF MODERN SCIENCE

(An award winning Research work on Homoeopathy)

Fifth fully Revised Edition
BY
Dr A.C.Dutta
&
Dr Swarup Dutta

Homoeopathy in the Light of Modern Science

First Edition: 1979

Second Edition: 1983

Third Edition: 1988

Fourth Edition: 1994

Preprint Edition: 1998

Fifth Completely revised and edited edition: 2020

ISBN: 9798740968230
Imprint: Independently published

(c) ALL RIGHTS RESERVED

DEDICATED

To all those who are fighting for salvation of science from orthodoxy.

Homoeopathy in the Light of Modern Science

CONTENTS

Publisher's Note
A Heart's Expression
Introduction
Acknowledgement
1. Evolution of Scientific Medical system
2. Emergence of Homoeopathy
3. High Dilution a Paradox?
4. Recent Researches
5. Concept of Vital Force
6. Modern Scientific Developments
7. A Scientific Look into the Process of Potentization
8. Modus Operandi
9. Chronic Miasm
10. Systematic of Prescribing
11. Homoeopathy in Cancer Treatment
12. Homoeopathy in Population Control
13. Homoeopathy in Plant Pathology
14. The Fate of Homeopathy in the Scientific World of 21st Century
15. Homeopathic Antibiotics?
16. Homoeopathy in pain management
17. Universal Scientific Recognition to Homoeopathy is inevitable
18. Homoeopathy a Light isotopic mode of Genetic Treatment

19. Frequently asked questions
    Conclusion
    Glossary
    References

TO BELIEVE SCIENCE DO WE NEED TO DISCARD OUR FAITH IN GOD AND SPIRITUALISM?

The question often asked is if science and spiritualism are co related? If one is scientific minded then should he stop believing in spiritualism and God?

I would like to answer this question with the help of a story which I read from somewhere:-

Once in a train, a man was sitting and reading a book while travelling. Another man entered the compartment and sat opposite to him. He could not stop himself and asked – what are you reading?

The man replied: "Bible"

The second man said ''I am surprised that you read the Bible in this era of science, where everything can be explained scientifically. Reading the Bible is just blind faith. What do you do for a living?'

The man replied – I am a scientist.

The second man was even more surprised. He said 'being a scientist how can you believe in all these things ?Please come and meet me and I will explain why these things are useless and has no base -Saying this he extended his business card to him.

Train reached the station.

Both men got down, The scientist asked the first man "I introduced myself to you, but you didn't introduce yourself"..

The first man gives his visiting card to the scientist, The scientist sees the card with eyes wide, printed on it was "**Thomas Alva Edison**". By that time Edison was already a well known name for his numerous inventions.

The scientist is surprised "Sir, please give your appointment. I want to come and see your laboratory."

Thomas gives appointment and they both meet in Thomas's lab,

In the lab there was a solar system model beautifully made by Thomas.

The scientist "The model looks beautiful, who made this?"

Thomas: Nobody, Yesterday it was not there- today it just appeared on its own"

The scientist gave a small snort of laugh and said "How is it possible? Jokes apart, Sir please tell me who made it?"

Edison insisted that it just appeared. The scientist retorted logically and scientifically speaking, it is impossible that it suddenly appeared.

Thomas: You are a scientist, you people say that suddenly one day the universe was created...Then how is not possible for this model to be created on its own??

Where there is a creation, there should be a creator, without a creator, there is no creation.

This brings us to the fundamental principle of Cause and effect- Where there is an effect there must be a cause.

If the universe we see exists then there should be a phenomenon which created it. If we try to trace the origin of anything you see in this world, you will end up either stagnating or getting in circles. A popular example in this context is that of the Chicken and the egg – which came first?

The problem with human beings is that we do not accept anything that does not fit into the block holes of our logic and intellect. We have become such slaves of our logic and intellect that doing so we are neglecting the entire universe. We have to clearly understand that there is much more in this universe which is beyond the grasp our silly intellect and cannot be perceived by human minds. The knowledge that we have acquired in the entire history of science is not even a size of a peanut compared to the ocean of knowledge that remains unexplored.

In this book we are talking about Quantum Physics and laws of Matter and energy. In the Vedic age the Rishis said' there is no difference between Shiva and Shakti - Shiva and Shakti are manifestations of the all-in-one divine consciousness - different sides of the same coin. Shiva symbolizes matter and Shakti symbolizes energy. Thousands of years later this same relation between energy and matter could be deduced and stated by the scientists.

The questions which remain unanswered are many; however an attempt has been made in this book to explain the scientific basis of Homoeopathy based on the discoveries of Modern science so far.

Homoeopathy in the Light of Modern Science

I request all readers to read the book with an open mind like that of a true scientist and not to accept or reject anything if it is not fitting in the block holes of your intellect. Neither the concept of Spirit like forces of Vital Force, potentization etc. is to be rejected. In this book we have tried to explain how energy and matter are interconvertible and how these concepts can be explained in the language of science and Homoeopathy.

Just like existence of God is not dependant on any evidence, the faith and need for God has kept Him alive in our hearts and minds, if Homoeopathy is a scientific mode of treatment or not ? Is a question that need not be answered. As long as patients will keep getting cured with this mode of treatment, it will stay alive in this world irrespective of what scientists have to say about it. However through this book, we have an answer to offer to the community of scientists and ask a question as well. The answer is 'Yes Homoeopathy is not only scientific but an extremely advanced science. Just like any other subject of science, it is based on countless trials and observations in different countries across different time. The question is simple- How long will you keep ignoring such an advanced science and pretend you cannot perceive its importance in the world of medical science? Don't behave like the young scientist who visited Edison's Laboratory and kept searching for the person who made the model of the universe ignoring the one who made the universe itself.

Let's accept the entire universe by understanding that it will not fit into the block holes of our intellect and it is perfectly ok to be that way. Just read the book to understand how Homeopathy can be explained with the help of Modern science and how Homeopathic medicines can bring about cure following the laws of this universe and nature.

Homoeopathy in the Light of Modern Science

"It is too naïve in asserting that theory should involve only observable magnitudes, but in fact it is theory that decides what is observable."

Albert Einstein

Homoeopathy in the Light of Modern Science

FATHER OF HOMOEOPATHY

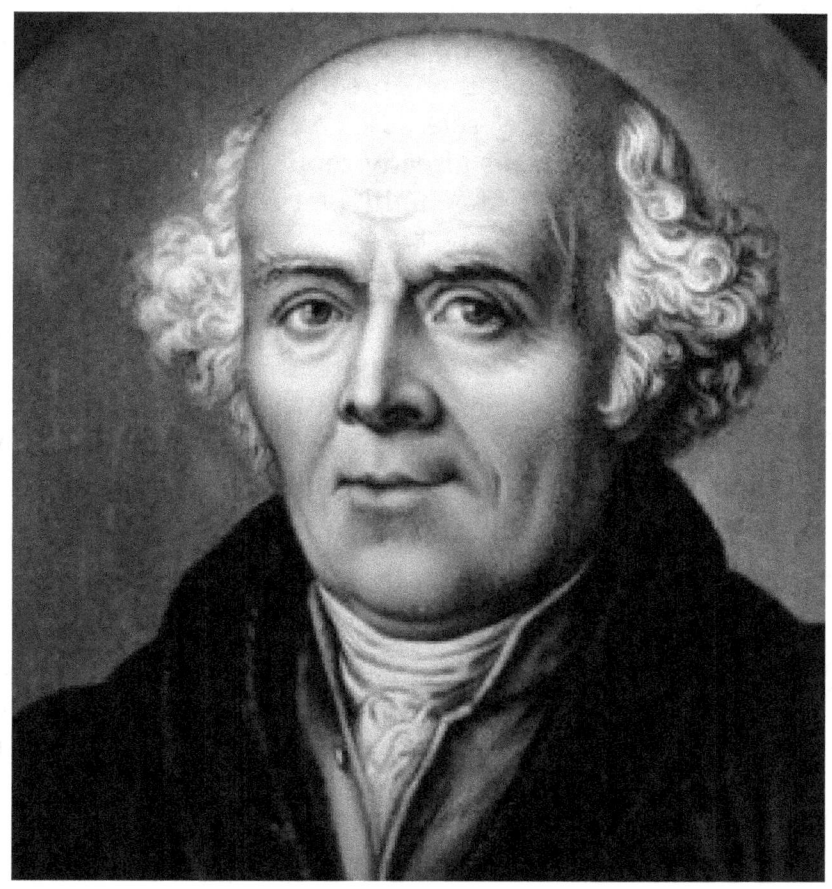

Dr. C.F. SAMUEL HAHNEMANN

10th April 1755 to 2nd July 1843

About the Authors

DR A.C. DUTTA (Homoeo- Scientist)

Dr. A.C.Dutta was born in the year 1936 in Jamshedpur, Bihar, India. A scientist by profession, Dr. Dutta was attached with a leading research institute of the country for more than three decades. Dr. Dutta, the propounder of the scientific basis of homoeopathic system of medicine, is already reputed nationally as well as internationally for his highly valuable contributions of scholarly scientific journals.

He is also the Founder Secretary of the International Centre for Cultivation of Homoeopathic Science (ICCHOS), Association for Advancement of Homoeopathic Science (AFAHS), author of 'Homoeopathic, a light isotopic treatment', Homeopathic treatment systematized and simplified and other books.

He was conferred the Yudhvir Singh Memorial award in 1995 and the Prestigious 'Mitra Award' in 1996 for postulating the missing link between Homoeopathy and Modern Science.

Dr A.C.Dutta is the first to propose the scientific basis of Homoeopathy based on Positronium complexes, way back in 1979. His work on drug standardization of Homoeopathic medicines was a path breaking research on Homoeopathic medicine as well.

DR SWARUP DUTTA (M.Sc; B.H.M.S, B.Ed)

Dr Swarup Dutta born in the year 1973 in Dhanbad, Bihar(now Jharkhand),India is the son of Dr A.C.Dutta.

He is an immensely versatile person and a very rare storehouse of experience in diverse fields –Scientific Research, Medicine, Education, Training, Manufacturing, Quality Management Systems, Business Management, Marketing, , Brand Management, Advertising, R&D, and Process building. He is a visionary leader and is presently working as a Principal in a CBSE affiliated school in Maharashtra (M.S.M English School and Junior College), he is also a master trainer and Zonal Coordinator of CBSE (Centre Of Excellence Pune). Recently his school has been selected by NITI Aayog for setting up Hi Tech STEM (Science Technology Engineering and Mathematics) Laboratory. He is equally passionate about Research in Homoeopathy and Education. Dr Swarup Dutta is the first school Principal in India to become a Master Black belt in Lean Six Sigma method of Quality Management system.

He is has more than 30 long years of experience in research with Dr A.C.Dutta and has been the closest companion of his father and participated in all scientific programs along with him since his school days. He grew up in a Research Institute Colony (C.F.R.I Colony) and came in contact with legendary Homeopaths like Dr Diwan Harish Chand, Dr Bholanath Chakraborty, Dr S.P.Dey, Dr Mahendra Singh and many others which helped him to develop and evolve as a true Homoeo – Scientist and Educator.

He is an orator par excellence, his speeches are extremely though provoking and directed to establish Homeopathy on solid scientific footings.

Publisher's Note

The importance and urgency of explaining homoeopathy in the light of modern science need not be stressed on. In this edition the authors have re-written the whole book in a popular from, so that it is easily understandable to the readers in general and the homoeopaths in particular.

We are sure that this new edition of the book will be received with much more enthusiasm than its predecessors.

A HEART'S EXPRESSION

Dated: 23.6.79

Dear Dr. Dutta,

The homoeopathic society as it stands today appears to care a fig for science and principles. They seem to be only after name and money, what to speak of bothering for the basic scientific problems, they even refuse to bother for the clinical aspects of homoeopathy, so far as the fundamental principles etc. are concerned with the sole mission of cure.

The only redeeming feature which is still sustaining my spirit is that a few people all over the world are coming forward to save homoeopathy from this most degrading situation and I deem you as one of them. And you will have to carry on with the valuable work that you are doing isolatedly, with the hope that the candle you are kindling will one day blaze out sufficiently to throw widespread light all over the medical world. And I also hope such a day is not very far off.

With best wishes,

Yours Sincerely,

J.N.Kanjilal

Excerpt from a letter of Late Dr. J.N.Kanjilal, a doyen and mentor of the homoeopathic profession and the then President of Honor of the HMAI.

Introduction

Application of a healing art without the science is generally regarded as a mere pretention and such practice is relegated to the domain of empiricism, Homoeopathic system of treatment, so far having no truck with the modern science, was never recognized as belonging to the category of scientific medicine. Rather it was often looked down as one of the worst quackeries that had ever come into existence.

Attempts have been, therefore, made in this treatise to find out the missing link between homoeopathy and the modern science. Reviewed in the light of some recent scientific discoveries, the doctrine of Homoeopathy, particularly its so-called darker sides, is found to be not only quite illuminative but also indicative of new vistas of research in the fields of micro-chemistry, micro-biology as well as plant pathology.

Not everything that exists (or does not exist) in this universe can be explained with the help of existing Science. There is much beyond the comprehension of human beings. However we attempt to explain things with whatever knowledge we have and if that is convincingly able to explain or predict the present and future actions, we are convinced of the explanation. This book convincingly resolves many questions raised on the scientificity of Homeopathy ,e.g – The potency phenomenon, the Concept of Vital Force, The Herring's Law of cure ,drug standardization of Homeopathic medicine, role of homoeopathic medicines in chronic diseases and will help the Homeopaths to answer these questions convincingly, most importantly it helps to approach other Homeopathic books like the Organon, Materia Medica, Pharmacy with a more scientific mind, so this is a must have book for every Homeopath and Homeopathic student.

A Few Comments Received

"You have written on a difficult but most important subject. A casual look shows the great efforts you have made."

Dr. Diwan Harish Chand
Ex. President, LMHI (Geneva)

"This is to acknowledge a complimentary copy of 'Homoeopathy in the Light of Modern Science'. Which I have read with great interest."

– Prof.V.Ramalingaswami
DG, ICMR (New Delhi)

"Your books were passed on to the centre's reading room in order that our visitors could also read them."

– Louissa Sossi
International Centre for Theoretical Physics (Italy)

"The author has given a sustained deep thought to find the scientific basis of the pathy. The hypothetical concepts presented are very appealing."

–Dr. K.P.Joshi
Reader in Physic (University of Indore)

"I have read your book with much interest. Your theory is quite comprehensive but its consequences would be revolutionary."

– Prof. S.C.Roy
R.E.College (Durgapur)

"Such persons who have command both in homoeopathy and modern science is a most disappointing rarely in our homoeopathic society. I sincerely wish all success in your mission."

– Dr.R.D.Mallick
Ex-President HMAI (W.B)

"I feel that by God's grace your sincere efforts will be fully crowned in near future. At least you will have the great consolation as Dr. Hahnemann had, who declared boldly- 'I have not lived in vain'."

– Dr. U.P.Dedhia
Bombay

Figures:

Some of the figures have been thankfully reproduced from the following books:

1. Transactions of the XXXII International Homoeopathic Medical Congress (New Delhi – 1977)
2. Hahnemann A Physician at the Dawn of New Era – by **Heinz Henne**
3. Biology – by **G.Padmanabhan** et al.
4. The Hahnemannian Gleanings, p.450, October 1976 (vol.XLIII,No.10) – by **J Boiron**
5. Homoeopathy a Light Isotopic Treatment – by **A.C.Dutta.**

Acknowledgement

The authors are indebted to Prof. S.R.Patil of the Indian Association for Cultivation of Science, and Dr. J. N. Kanjilal, a doyen and mentor of homoeopathic profession in India, for their kind advices and support.

We are immensely grateful to Dr Diwan Harish Chand for his tremendous support and appreciation and for his role to propagate the scientific basis of Homoeopathy mentioned in this book. The 'Mitra award' given to Dr A.C.Dutta in 1996 was under his patronage.

The authors are also grateful to the colleagues of Dr.A.C.Dutta, Scientists of C.F.R.I (Now C.I.M.F.R), many homeopaths and a few close relatives who extended their whole hearted support and co-operation in establishing the scientific basis of Homoeopathy.

Thanks are particularly due to Mrs Minati Dutta, Wife of Dr A.C.Dutta, because without her active co-operation it would have been really difficult to present this work. Incidentally she is also the first publisher of the book.

Dr Bisakha Dutta, wife of Dr Swarup Dutta and their son Soham Dutta have been extremely supportive and a constant source of motivation.

Mrs Manisha Majumder, daughter of Dr A.C. Dutta, Jayabrata Majumder (son in law) & Arkadeep Majumder

(grandson) needs to be thanked as well for their loving support.

The author is thankful to Dr P.G. Mohata (M.B.B.S, D.C.H) for his constant support and encouragement. His spiritual insights have been extremely valuable in the life of Dr Swarup Dutta and his entire family.

The author extends his heartfelt thanks to Sri D.G.Mahajan, Sri Govind Baheti and all the members of Gauri Shankar Seva Samity and of M.S.M Family for their constant motivation and support.

Finally the authors are grateful to all the readers of this book for devoting their time for the cause of Homoeopathic science

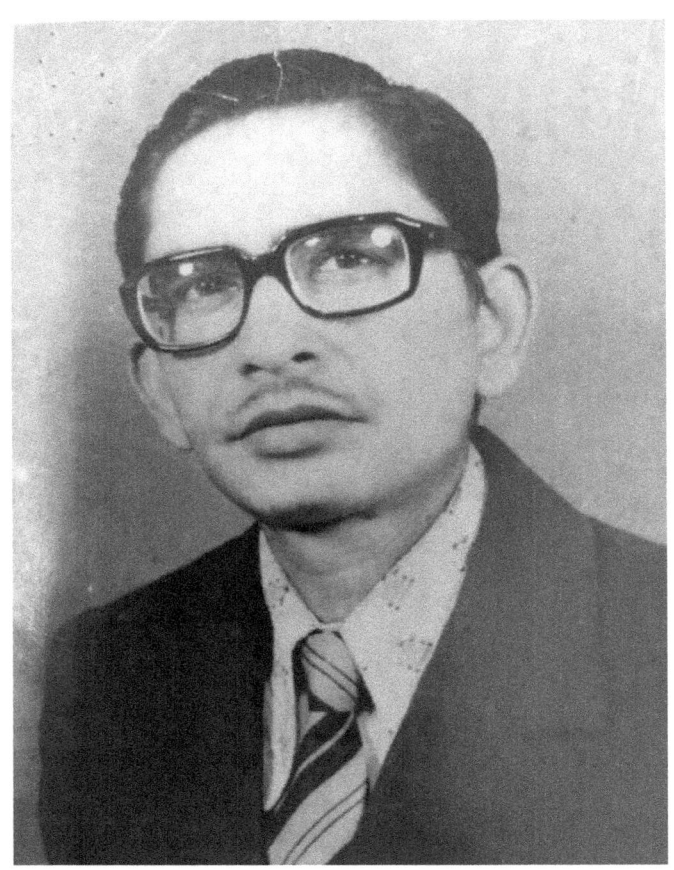

Dr.A.C.Dutta
Scientist
1936-2019

1. Evolution of Scientific Medical System

Medical treatment among primitive people was either magical or purely empirical. It included application of heat and cold, bloodletting, counter irritation, baths, suction, etc. The pharmacopoeia included purgatives and emetics, but consisted mostly of herbal substances without physiological action. It also included substances of disgusting character, the use of which was based on the belief that it would discomfort the possessing spirit and consequently the latter would vacate the body of its victim.

The first rational or scientific medical system was Greek, exhibited from about 500 B.C. till the rise of the Roman Empire. Much of the Hippocratic !collection, which contains the earliest as well as the best Greek medical writings, was put together in the 4th century B.C.

During the 16th and the first half of the 17th centuries anatomy and physiology had put on their modern dress. Andreas Vesalius (1514-1564), the father of modem anatomy, was worthy successor of Leonardo da Vinci. Sanctorius (1561-1636) laid the foundation of the study of metabolism. Jerome Fabricius (1537-1619) was the founder of modern embryology and William Harvey (1578-1657) was the discoverer of the blood circulation, the basis of the whole of the modern rational medicine. In 1546 Girolamo Fracastoro set forth a rational theory of infection that had superficial resemblance to the germ doctrine. Guillaume de Baillon (1538-1616) contributed to the conception of epidemics by introducing the Hippocratic idea of 'epidemic constitution' which further developed under Thomas Sydenham (1624- 1689) and still has value'.

The 18th century dawned with the refreshing breeze of Newtonian philosophy blowing through it and **the new generation was apparently bewildered with the** novelty and mass of the material.

The first half of the century exhibits something **of a gap** in the progress **of** research, particularly in **the medical** field and **excepting** Boerhaave (1668- **1738) and** Haller (1708-1777) **there** was none to fill **up the** void. **Boerhaave was the** first clinical **or** 'bedside'- **teacher and Haller** did some **work on mechanical** respiration, **formation of** bone, **action of** digestive **juice etc.**

During the 18th century, the practice of the physicians remained largely medieval and the ruling idea was still humoral .In fact science of internal medicine lagged behind surgery, because anatomical reforms of Vesalius had no counterpart to advance physiological knowledge. No fundamental new principle was however introduced in surgery. The theories of diseases were still speculative and better apparatus for diagnosis were lacking.

At the turn of the 20th century, there were only a few drugs and other measures of outstanding importance, some of which **being** improperly understood. Although **the** foundation for its development was laid in the earlier years, the modem therapeutics followed World War-1.

Homoeopathy in the Light of Modern Science

The doctrine of the essential cellular nature (Figure 1.2 to1.4) of living beings had been established by 1840 and the conception of protoplasm (Figure **1.1)** as the 'physical basis of life' came into clear view. The study of tissues histology—-was raised to the status of an independent science by Albert von Kolliker (1817-1905) and a very important influence on medical thought was achieved by Rudolf Virchow **(1821-** 1902) when he extended the cell conception to diseased tissues.

In 1912, Casimir Funk introduced the term 'Vitamin' to designate accessory food factors which arc required in the diet in small amounts. Since then many of these substances were identified, their chemical structures determined and synthesis achieved.

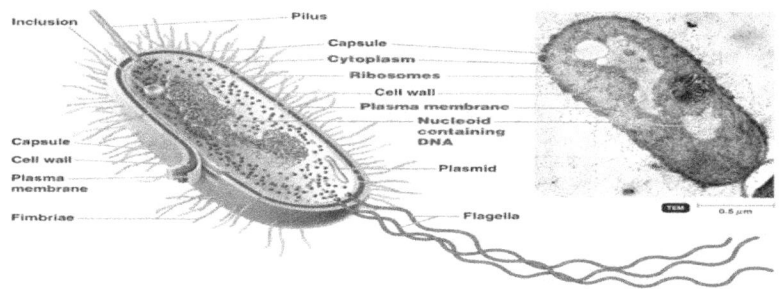

Figure 1.2   Components of a bacterium

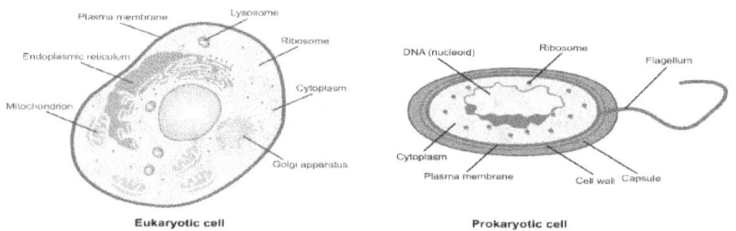

Figure 1.3   A cell under ordinary microscope

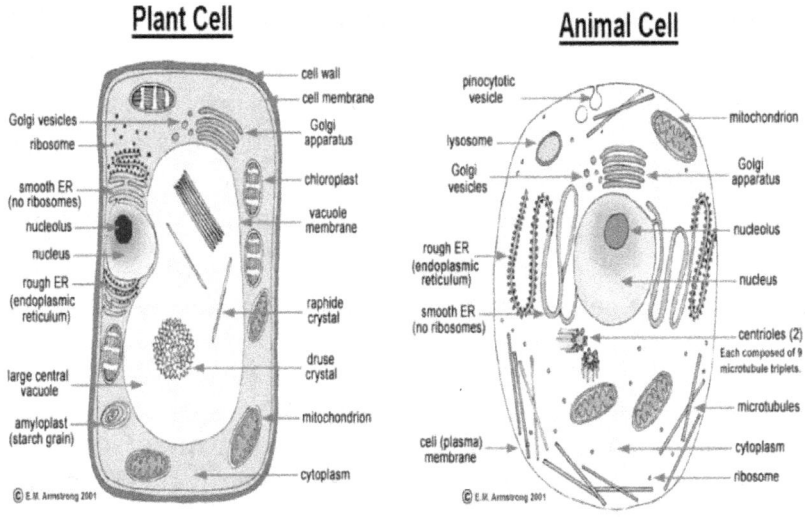

Figure 1.4 Diagrammatic comparison of (A) Plant cell (B) Animal cel

BACTERIA CELL ANATOMY

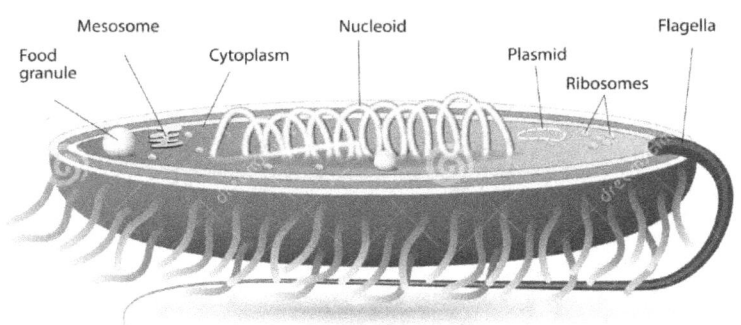

Figure 1.5 Flagellate to a bacteria

The germ doctrine of diseases (Figure 1.2 & 1.5) advanced by Louis Pasteur (1822-1853) and Robert Koch (1843-1910) was, however, the centre of the triumphs of medicine during the last hundred years although received by the conservatives with skepticism and even hostility, it created a revolution in medical thought and still remain the basis of the whole concept of prevention and cure of many communicable diseases.

Within the period 1871 to 1884, the organisms responsible for leprosy, gonorrhoea, tuberculosis, typhoid, Cholera, Diphtheria etc. were known. By 1888, it was generally realized that the symptoms of diseases were the result of the poisonous substances produced by the action of the organisms and the substances were specific for many forms. The word 'toxin' was introduced to describe them.

Although Edward Jenner (1796) had preached the prevention of small pox by the inoculation of humans with cow pox, it was Louis Pasteur, who really enunciated the philosophy of vaccination against bacterial and even viral infection. In 1888, preventive vaccination against typhoid fever was introduced and in 1894, the method of inducing 'passive immunity' was successfully used and later on widely adopted.

All these work were, however, contemporary with the rise of the new surgical technique, especially connected with the name of Joseph Lister (1822- 1912). In 1846 'anesthesia' was introduced but great developments in surgery were possible only after 1930.

In 1922 Alexander Fleming discovered 'penicillin'.

This proved to be efficacious in treating a wide variety of infections including pneumonia, sub acute endocarditis, syphilis, gonorrhoea etc. Soon a whole field of investigations sprang up in which systematic search was made for antibacterial or antiviral substances produced by other organisms.

Many of the important advances in medicine tern from developments in fields apparently unrelated to medicine, such as physics, chemistry, electronics etc.

Following the basic chemical and physical findings m the 19th century, modem chemotherapy and therapeutics were born, which in turn was it responsible for the development of huge drug industries. In addition to the general laboratory techniques, new diagnostic instruments were perfected. Radiology, angiocardiography, tissue culture, blood transfusion etc. came into practice.

After the discovery of radio-active isotopes in 1934 by F.J. and I.J. Curie it began to be applied in biological problems and had a great influence on the course of medical research.

But after the marathon race of nearly hundred years, the whole of the medical world seems today set aback, particularly by the adverse influences of many of its highly acclaimed modern medicines.

No one argues now that vaccine damage does not exist. In fact more and more reports are available on children being seriously injured as a result of routine immunization amounting even to total blindness, dumbness, deafness and epilepsy.

Indiscriminate use of antibacterial drugs has also exacted a heavy toll throughout the world. Mishaps following the light-hearted prescription and supply of other drugs are also reported.

After more than 30 years, doctors bombarding gonococci with increasing quantities of penicillin, their principal weapon against gonorrhoea that tops the list of world's communicable diseases, now the penicillin-resistant gonorrhoea is in picture. Possibility of dangerous meningococcus and other organisms becoming penicillin resistant are also feared[4]. Severe restrictions have already been imposed on the promotion and recommended use of some potentially harmful drugs, such as thalidomide, chloramphenicol etc[5].

Today it is observed that for all its achievements in 40 years of booming growth, the drug industry is failing to meet many of the needs of the poor majority of the world population. The question is also being raised about the ability of the industry to produce safe drugs[6].

Further, observations have even been made that the medical establishment has become a major threat to health[6], and that the pharmaceutical industry may not be nearly so vital to our well-being in the years ahead as it has been in the recent past[5].

2. Emergence of Homoeopathy

Samuel Hahnemann, the founder of homoeopathy, was born on April 10th 1755, in Meissen on Elbe in Germany. His father Christian Gottfried used his creative talents as a certified painter of porcelain. Hahnemann later remembered proudly his father's fine practical senses.

After having attended the local school, Hahnemann entered the reputed school at St. Afra, wherefrom he received an excellent education in the areas of classical and modern languages. He is said to have read the writings of Hippocrates while at this school. In later life he further advanced on the famous Hippocratic concept that diseases might be cured either by opposites or similar by his theory of 'Similia Similibus Curentur' (let likes be cured by likes).

He began to study medicine in Leipzig in 1775. In the spring of 1777 Hahnemann found his way to Vienna at his own expense, because of his love of practical pharmacology. In Vienna school of that time the intense interaction between the renaissance of Hippocratism and the tendencies of enlightened medicine was achieved, which was very important for medicine of the 18th century[7].

A de Haen, the Director of the Vienna school was fully aware of the limitations of medical knowledge. From the very beginning he perceived it his chief duty to free the medical profession from its 'many superfluous doctrines', and unnecessary trifles so that these would not become harmful to either the patients or the physicians. Hahnemann was also deeply influenced by a Vienna physician Plenciz, who was highly revered at that time for his scientific achievements. The conviction of Plenciz that diseases are produced by lower organisms remained with him all his life[7].

On August 10th 1779, the degree of Doctor of Medicine was conferred upon him by the University of Erlangen (Figure 2.1). In 1781 Hahnemann was called to Gommern to become district medical officer. In the following year he married Henriette, step-daughter of the apothecary Haseler in Dessau, and hoped to be able to live in a state of financial security from then on.

But his overly sensitive conscience made him think that his treatment of sick people had often done more harm than good. For so often physicians had to grope around in the dark and afterwards treat an unknown state of a disease, the symptoms of which might or might not be real, with remedies whose specific effect might be unknown, or at best only received their classification in the material medica at someone's discretion.

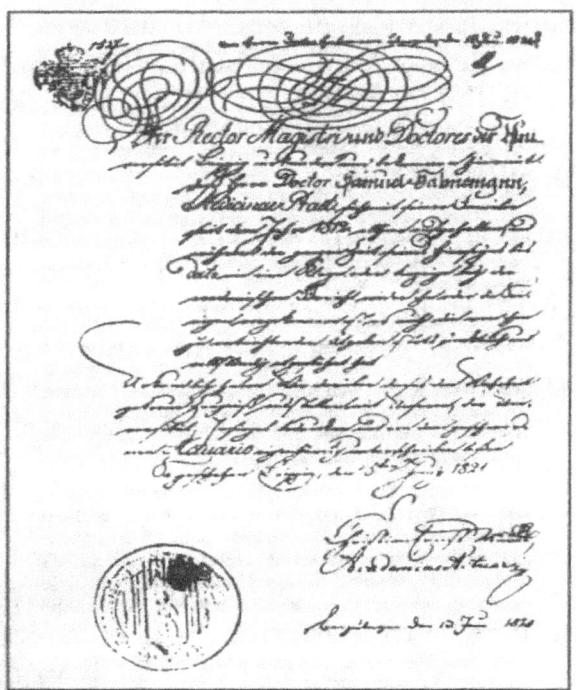

Figure 2.1

Copy of Medical certificate issued by Hahnemann

Potent substances, if not entirely suited to the patient, would certainly cause harm, in the form of new pains and chronic ailments which are more difficult to relieve than the original disease. The average doctors of course would not inform his patient of this danger[7].

The physician had a flood of information about the newest chemical and natural preparations, but he did not know to which specific case of a disease they were suited and where they would provide reliable aid. These cases were almost totally unknown on the part of the pharmacist. Only overlapping and often contradictory presumptions about many remedies were known.

So as a young man Hahnemann had to convince himself 'in stages' that "the art of healing was on the wrong path". He no longer wanted to serve a profession which was harmful to humanity. During the first years of his marriage, he almost totally abandoned his practice and concerned himself with chemistry and writing.

It is interesting to note Hahnemann recalling in later age that the famous 'truth-loving' C. Hufeland had told him that he divided his patients into three categories: Those which Nature would have healed more quickly than he, those which Nature would have healed as well as he, and those in which he assisted Nature in doing the job[7].

In 1790, while translating W. Cullen's materia medica, Hahnemann contradicted Cullen's observa-tion that 'Cinchona bark' helps in the case of intermittent fever because it is bitter and a 'tonic for the stomach'. He objected that the quick antipyretic effect of the cinchona bark administered immediately prior to an attack could not be explained in that way. The bark had been applied to a considerable degree and helped randomly or did damage.

He was concerned with proving on which kind of intermittent fever cinchona bark always had an effect. For the sake of the experiment he took four grains of good cinchona twice daily for several days. Only after repeating this dosage did till the 'normal symptoms of intermittent fever' appear, one after another, but without tremors.

Thus Hahnemann was able to form his judgment on intermittent fever and its treatment with cinchona bark. Furthermore, he pointed out that substance like Arsenic that are able to cause a kind of fever, are also capable of alleviating this in the patient.

Thus, as he could be convinced at that time, Hahnemann's 'new principle' similia similibus had taken shape through experimentation and experience.

Hahnemann took a moderate stand on the matter without making a precise reference in his "Essay on a new principle to determine the healing powers of medicinal substances, including consideration of those to date", published in 1796 in Hufeland's journal. He explained that chemistry could not simply be banned from medicine.

In early 19th century Hahnemann through his famous books, 'The Organon of Medicine' (1810) and 'On Chronic Diseases' (1825) established the epoch- making new system of treatment called "Homoeopathy". The new system of treatment introduced by him proved to be revolutionary and received wide acceptance throughout the world (Figure 2.2). It enjoyed great influence and success till the 1880's and thereafter for various reasons it experienced some setback, particularly in advanced western countries. Incidentally the then existing system of dominant

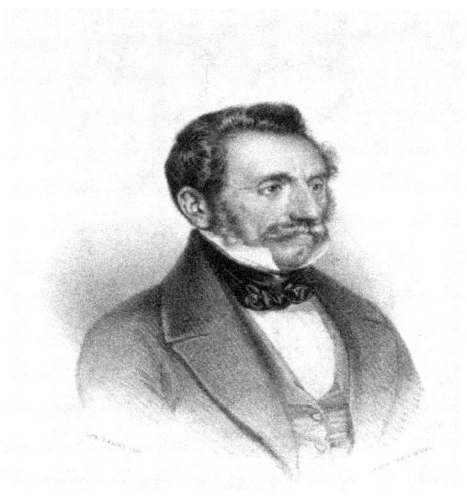

Figure 2.2(a) Dr. Johann Martin Honigberger
Who first brought homoeopathy to India

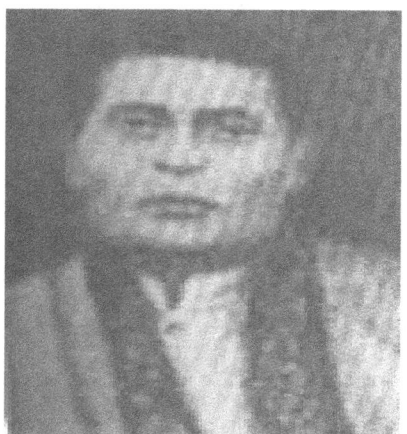

Figure 2.2 (b)
Rajendra Lal Dutta *Father of Indian homoeopathy*

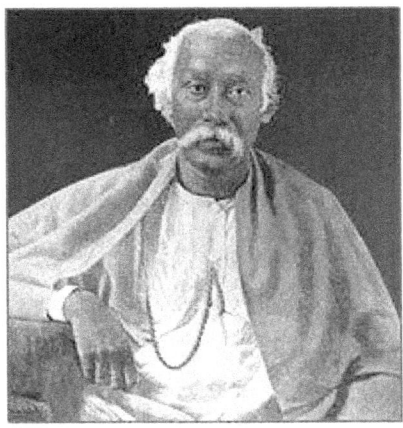

Figure 2.2 (c)

Dr Mahendra Lal Sirkar

A scientist and allopathic physician who took big role in advancing Homoeopathy in India.

School of medicine was named by Hahnemann as 'Allopathy' as opposed to homoeopathy.

It is not difficult to imagine the negative reaction of both apothecaries and many contemporary physicians who condemned Hahnemann's empirical viewpoints as too radical and unrealistic. Hahnemann was said to have been driven on from one place to another by the apothecaries.

Hahnemann's use of insignificantly small doses of medicine was also a matter of ridicule. By the year 1800 Hahnemann had made frequent use of greatly diluted medicines. Initially intended to get rid of the toxic adverse effects of the drug substances as far as possible, soon he was convinced of the much higher efficacy of such greatly diluted remedies.

In his 'Organon', he established the general principle concerning dosage, that in opposition to the hitherto existing practice, one should administer an appropriate medicine in such a dose as would only just suffice to achieve the intended results, and not affect the body unnecessarily.

But later on he professed in his work 'On chronic diseases' that it indeed took a lot of self conviction to believe that such an "incredibly small" medicinal dose could have an effect for many weeks. He did not demand that anyone believe him and did not expect this to be conceivable to anyone. He himself could not conceive of it either. But it was the absolute fact and experience that confirmed it was so.

In regard to his therapeutic observations he raised a question in his characteristic manner, "Do we not want to imitate an action until the wonderful natural forces underlying it are brought before our very eyes and explained to us in a child-like fashion? Would it not be idiotic not to want to make fire with steel and stone because one cannot conceive how such boundless energy can be stored up in these materials?".

3. High Dilution A Paradox

Hahnemann, the propounder of the theory of 'similia similibus Curentur' developed concurrently a special process of dilution for use in homoeopathic system of medicine, which created great deal of controversy.

The process was known to be effected by mechanical action upon the smallest portions of the drug substances by means of rubbing or shaking, through the addition of an inert (non-medicinal) substance, powder or liquid, e.g. sugar of milk or alcohol and in a series[8]. The process was thus known as 'dynamizing' or 'potentizing' and the products were called 'potencies' in different degrees.

Detailed method of preparation is as follows: One drop of the drug substance is put in a vial i.e small cylindrical glass vessel. To this are added ninety-nine drops of pure alcohol, when the vial is two-third filled. Stoppered with a velvet cork, ten violent shakings (succussions) are then given to the vial against a hard but elastic body, with hand or machine. Thus homoeopathic remedy of first degree of dynamization or one centesimal (1c) potency is prepared.

One drop of this 1 c potency is then taken into a fresh vial, mixed with fresh ninety-nine drops of alcohol (ethanol) and fresh ten successive strokes are given, when '2C' potency is said to be produced. Thus the process is repeated until 3c, 6c, 30c, 200c or still higher potencies are obtained.

Alternatively, the insoluble drug substances are known to be prepared by rubbing (triturating) rather strongly and in a specific manner, one part of the drug substance mixed with nine parts of sugar of milk using a mortar-pestle and a spatula, each made of porcelain. The degree of potentization thus obtained is said to be in the decimal level and are marked as lx, 2x, 6x, 12x, etc.

The process however involved a great deal of mysticism, which became all the more apparent with the resurrection of Avogadro's hypothesis in 1860. As per Avogadro's number, the number of molecules in a gram-molecular weight (molecular weight expressed in gram) of any substance is 6.06×10^{23} (roughly twenty-four naughts after one).

During the early twentieth century the hypoth-esis was repeatedly verified and confirmed through various experiments by J. Perrin (1909), B. B. Boltwood and E. A. Rutherford (1911), R. A. Millikan (1917) and R. T. Birge (1941). They all found that the Avogadro's number stands good, only a minor correction was necessary. Instead of 6.06×10^{23}, it should be 6.023×10^{23}.

This shook the very basis of the homoeopathic system of dilution, making thereby the whole system of medicament unacceptable to the scientific world. Because on projection of the Avogadro's hypothesis to the homoeopathic system of dilution, it was found that once the 12th centesimal or 24th decimal homoeopathic dilution is surpassed, there cannot exist any atom or molecule of the original drug substance.

To be more precise the molecular weight of Ferrum Metallicum being 55.85. or the molecular weight of sodium chloride i.e. Natrum Muriaticum being 58.44 or that of the molecular weight of Aurum Metallicum i.e. metallic gold being 107.0, therefore 55.85 grams of

Ferrum Metallicum. or 58.44 grams of Natrum Muriaticum or 107.0 grams of Aurum Metallicum contain a fixed number of molecules of the respective substances being 6.023x 10^{23} (roughly twenty-four zeros after one).

Now if we start preparing homoeopathic medicines with the same quantity, while going to 2c potency from 1 c potency, we will have to take only one part out of hundred, which will contain hundredth part of original number of molecules (i.e. twenty-two zeros after one). In the next potency it will be again hundredth part of that of the previous potency (i.e. twenty zeros after one) and so on. (Figure 3.1)

Thus at every higher potency two zeros being eliminated, once the 12c potency is reached there

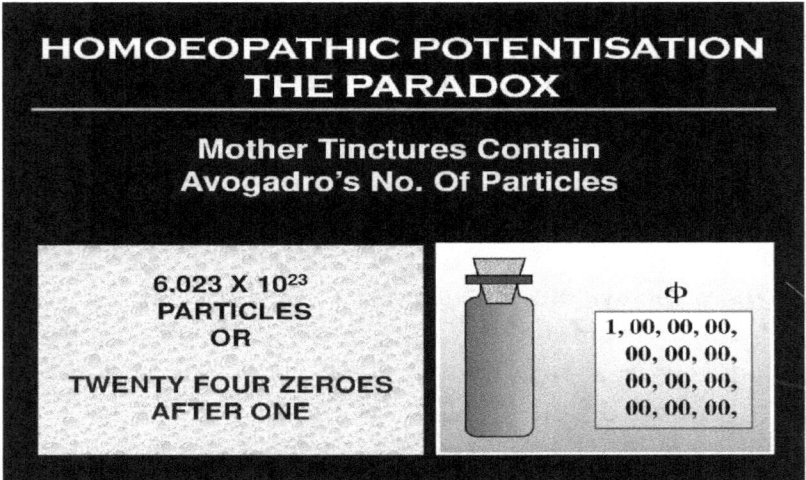

Figure 3.1

The mother tincture (Q) and also 1 c potency contain a large number of drug molecules

Homoeopathy in the Light of Modern Science

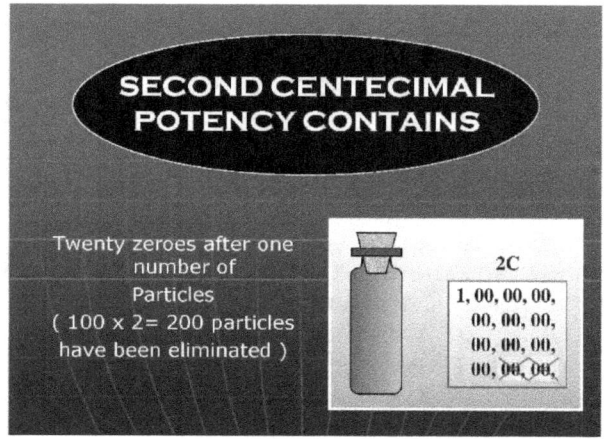

Figure 3.2 *In the process of serial dilution, after 12c potency practically all drug molecules are eliminated.*

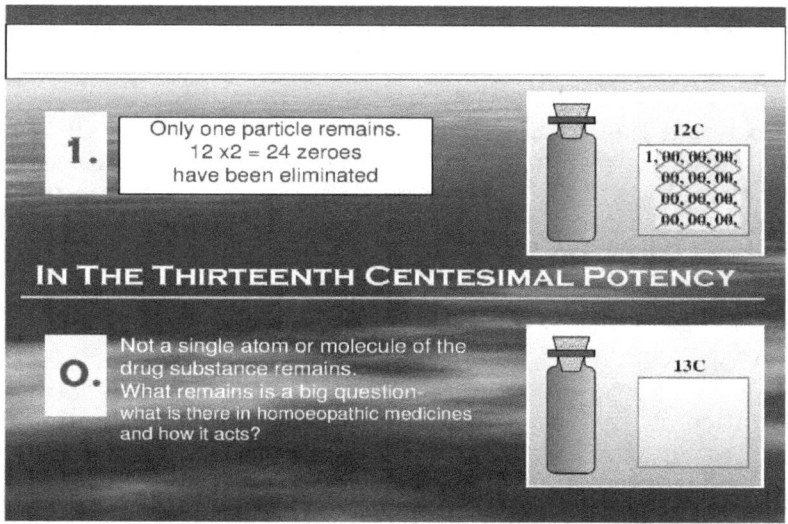

Figure 3.3 *30c and higher potencies contain absolutely no drug*

molecule. The Question remains – 'how it works then?'

will be no molecule of the original drug substances present. In case of decimal potency as at every stage only one zero is to be eliminated, such condition is expected to reach once the 24x potency is surpassed (Figures 3.2 & 3.3).

This mathematical conclusion was also found to be true on various instrumental observations such a High Performance Liquid Chromatography (HPLC), Gas Liquid Chromatography (GLC), Atomic Absorption Spectro-photometer (AAS), Ultraviolet Spectroscope (UVS) etc. when no molecule of the original drug substances could be traced after the 12c or 24x homoeopathic potencies.

Even on probability consideration it becomes, therefore, difficult to conceive scientifically the presence of any molecule of the original drug substance in the homeopathically administered does of as low homoeopathic dilution as 30c. Such preparations are therefore thought to be simple 'ethanol' or 'water', having no therapeutic value.

Science has established beyond a shadow of doubt that matter is not infinitely divisible and molecules are the ultimate units of transaction in any chemical or bio-chemical reaction. So any dilution of matter to a stage where hardly a unit of atom or molecule is likely to be encountered in a given does of medicine, loses all meaning in scientific sense.

Moreover, as per the well established, 'Law of Mass Action', it is known that the chemical action of a reacting substance is proportional at any moment to its 'active mass' or in other words its 'molecular concentration'. In this background it is also difficult to hold scientifically the homoeopathic claim that 'higher the homoeopathic dilution stronger the medicine'.

Confronted with this awkward situation various attempts were made at different times to interpret

Homoeopathy in the Light of Modern Science

homoeopathic system of dilution corroborating with modern scientific concepts.

Hahnemann himself in this connection observed that several changes are known to be brought about in different natural substances by means of friction, such as development of heat, development of odour in odourless bodies, magnetization of steel bar and so forth. A steel bar is unable to draw magnetically or hold on either end even finest particles of iron. But when dynamized by rubbing it with a magnetic bar in one direction, it soon becomes a true active powerful magnet, able to attract iron and steel to itself and impart to another bar of steel the magnetic power and this in a higher degree the more it has been rubbed. In the same way, Hahnemann believed that by triturating a medicinal substance and/or by shaking vigorously its solution, the medicinal powers hidden within it is more and more developed and manifested[8]

In recent-times, however, knowing fully well that the atoms and molecules of substances, the ultimate units of transaction in chemistry, meet quickly the Avogadrian impasse, in the process of serial dilution and succussion (potentization), more plausible explanations were put forward.

In the beginning it was thought that the added kinetic energy in the process of succussion is retained in the vehicle, thereby causing the molecules to be more potent or energetic[10]. But soon it was realized that the kinetic/mechanical energy will fairly rapidly get converted into thermal energy and consequently the energetic state of molecules will be short-lived and the normal molecular modes will be restored as the heat energy get decayed.

Thereafter it was proposed that the potency phenomenon should better be viewed entropically rather than energetically[11]. Entropy is said to be a measure of the heat that flows during a thermodynamic process or of the information that is transmitted during a communicating process. Change of entropy is known to indicate changes of unavailable energy in a system that may generally occur by addition or subtraction of heat or by frictional processes in the system.

During frictionless process with no heat added or abstracted the entropy is said to be zero. It was therefore proposed that the change of entropy through the successive process involved in homoeopathic system of dilution is responsible for the specific information transmission. The entropic model for homoeopathic potencies, however, failed to explain why at the same potency level, different homoeopathic medicines can act differently.

Then it was proposed that the potency phenomenon should better be explained through the 'cybernetic' (communication) models. Cybernetics is known to be the science of control and communication in all of its various manifestations in machines, animals and organisations. The term was first introduced by the mathematician Norbcrt Wiener in a book called 'cybernetics', published in 1948.

Contrary to most other sciences, the transfer of energy is usually of little consequence and transfer of information is said to be the vital in cybernetics. The cybernetic model for homoeopathic potency, however, ultimately failed to explain the significance of the term 'dynamization' or 'potentisation' and these were proposed to be substituted by the term 'succussed dilution' as nothing was believed to be made more powerful in the process[10].

Further, in the homoeopathic system of dilution, as the vehicle (ethanol) constitutes the only continuum between the low and the high dilutions, it was proposed that the therapeutic activity of homoeopathic dilutions lie in the structure itself of the vehicle, in the form of specific arrangement of the ethanol molecules between themselves[11].

The admission of a fresh supply of air, containing the non-polar oxygen molecules, at each stage of serial dilution, followed by impacted succussion was said to function as 'informational templates' of the original drug molecules, transmitting the same from lower to higher dilution.

The over-simplified proposition could not be accepted, because the chemical properties of sub-stances are said to depend on the internal electronic arrangement of the atoms of the molecules and not on the external molecular orientation of the substances. Further it raised the questions as to the actual role of oxygen in the process of succussion and also the nature of interactions between the respective biological system and the specific liquid structure.

Thus the propositions put forward to interpret 'the scientific basis of homoeopathic system of dilution not only found to be lacking in universally acceptable data but also appeared to be mere speculative.

4. Recent Researches

In chemistry, there is no special technique related to homoeopathy. Microchemistry, chromatography or even capillary spectra can reach the limit of the sensibility around a dilution 10^{-7} or 10^{-8} which are very much within the Avogadro's limit.

Therefore, the Homoeo-scientists mainly concentrated to physical methods. In 1933 Loch built an apparatus named the Microlyometer for the demonstration of the presence of matter in dilutions and to establish the curves of these dilutions.

In 1936 W.E. Boyd of Glasgow, published the results of his research made with spectrograph. There the sensibility limit was found to reach only the 7th decimal for Aurum, Arsenicum and China. 7th decimal represents in current language a solution of 1/1,000,000,0 which is in fact rather a concentrated solution compared to homoeopathic dilution[12].

At about the same time, O. Lesser and K. Janner published their research with radioactive phosphorus. They found the limit dosages at the 18th decimal (or 9th centesimal) dilution.

Heinz studied the physical action of dilutions using the infra-red spectra and stressed on the specific value of succussion. Like Gay, he found the rhythmicity indicating some favourable points in the curve of dilution.

Gay and J.Boiron (1951-1952) made a series of studies (Figure 4.1) and gave results obtained with Gay's montage named the 'gayograph'. However, it was observed, in their delicate measurement certain variations could be produced by the glass solubility or by the use or corks[12].

Physical researches include also those of Dr. Sevaux et al, who checked the unpublished experiments of Mr. Vojn Radojicie regarding measurements of copper sulphate solution from 1st to 20th decimal potency (10th centesimal). They used bio electrometer of Vincent.

Although chemical or physical methods were used to trace the presence of matter in dilution, yet it was believed that the link between the matter in dilution and the activity of these dilutions could be best achieved by biological methods. Since by reciprocity these methods enable one to detect the presence of a given substance by the activity of the product under investigation.

Raulin, Charles Richet, Gabriel Bertrand and Javillier were first who demonstrated the role of oligoelements, so-called biocatalyst, on the growth of Aspergillus niger or on yeasts(Silver,Zinc,Manganese), and on the laccase activity(manganese). Of course these experiments are not homoeopathic but they are often cited by the homoeopaths to prove the reality or action of infinitesimal doses.

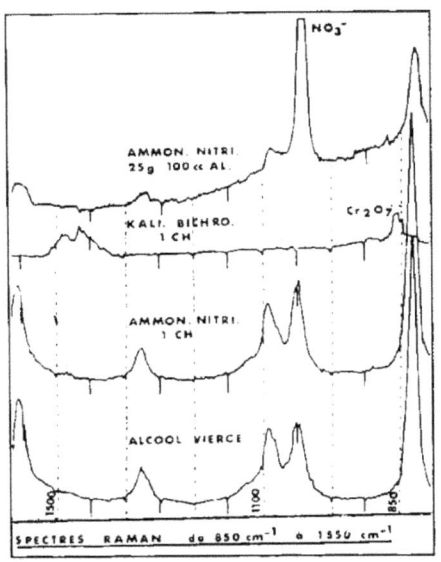

Figure 4.1(a)

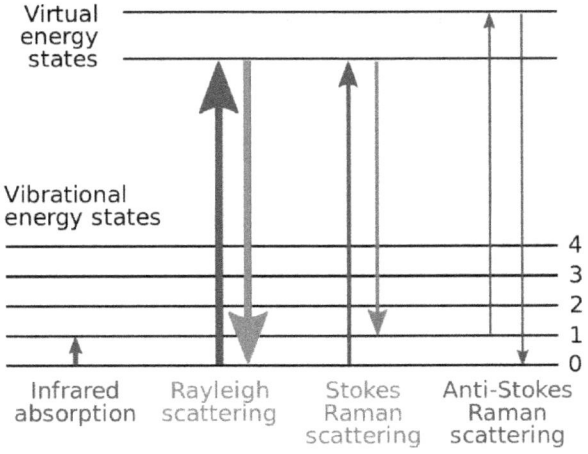

Figure 4.1(b)

W.E. Persson studied the influence of micro doses of Iris, Phosphoric acid end Arsenic on the diastatic action of trypsine. With successive dilutions a sinusoidal curve was found.

Dr. Nebel in in 1932 experimented on yeasts, intoxicated by Merc. Cor. Arndt and Schulz also experimented on yeast with Merc.cor. Iodine, Bromium and Salicylic acid and showed that in the weak doses these substances increase the multiplication of yeasts, yet strong doses kill them. More recently, Prof. Netien et al studied the action of infinitesimal dilution of Naturm arsenicosum on the growth of yeasts in functions of these dilutions.

Dr. Lamasson studied the action of Korsakovian dilutions up to the 'M' on cultures of staphylococcus aureus. Hinsdale showed the inhibitive action of Calendula on staphylococcus.

Trying to demonstrate the desensitizing action of Apis mel. Dr. Doneche used white rats injected intra-peritoneally with ovalbumin solution. Apis 3rd centesimal or 5th centesimal injected at the same time as the ovalbumin, and then every half an hour, lessened considerably the oedema. J. and M. Telau observed that the diluted doses of Thuja disturbed the psychic balance of rats which lose their conditioning.

Various works were also reported to be conducted with high dilutions on the vegetable realm. Of course few are the works that related to homoeopathy, and undoubtedly many results need to be confirmed.

Mrs. Kolisko (1926) made considerable studies on effects of high dilution on young plants' growth. She demonstrated the action of dilution up to the 60th decimal or even beyond to the 200th decimal. She also observed the rhythmic and sinusoidal curve. Prof. Netien also studied the action of cobalt in homoeopathic dilutions on the breathing of wheat coleoptyle[12].

In recent time the authors conducted a good number of experiments on wheat seeds, germinated in distilled water culture grown under the effect of high dilution of some known 'macro' and 'micro nutrients' such as Ferrum sulphuricum, Cuprum sulphuricum etc. It was found that while by post germination treatment of the substances, by dilutions even beyond the Avogadro's limit, considerable growth stimulation effect were observed, by pre germination treatment specific disease symptoms in plants were produced. The disease symptoms were found to be more prominent in higher dilution i.e. 1M potency than in lower dilution i.e. 6c potency.

With the discovery of micronutrients, a large number of hitherto obscure, plant diseases were identified as micro-nutrient deficiencies. But it became difficult to reconcile how the similar disease symptoms could be developed by the substances in toxic level.

Dr. Nebel conducted several experiments on entire animal. He had been, however, censured for using too few animals. So his experiments have not been duplicated However, he tried several approaches: a 30th or 200th decimal dilution of mallein injected three weeks after injection of a live culture in the ear of a rabbit produced an intense vasodilation of the peritumoral vessels while the opposite ear, intact, did not react at all.

Arthus studied the action of Calc. fluor in rickets. One per cent of Calc.fluor in 3rd decimal potency prolonged the life of rats as compared with controls submitted to the same rachitogenic diet. Hofmeister studied the action of Pulsatilla on the genital function of the while mice (Figure 4.2). He however stated that it was not comparable with that of the action of hormones.

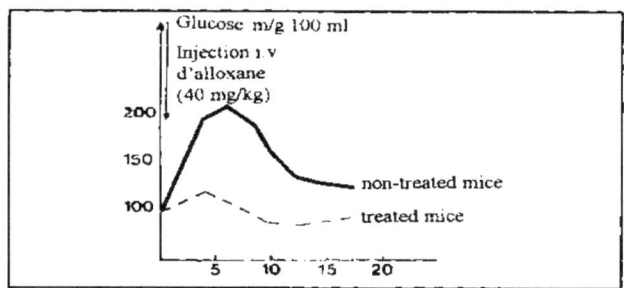

Figure 4.2

Dr. Cantegrit tried to show the euphylactic effects of a high dilution of Nux vomica in a guinea pig intoxicated with strychnine'. Martiny and Pretec studied the anaphylactic phenomena.

Dr. Jarricot studied the action of veratrine on the muscular contraction of the frog gastrocnemius and concluded that a 30th Korsakovian dilution favours the work of the muscle. He then studied the action of Iberis amara on the isolated heart of frog or tortoise.

In recent time the French biologist Jacques Benveniste published in 'Nature' (1988) a paper titled "Human basophil degranulation triggered by very dilute antiserum against Ig E". The paper created lot of controversy in the scientific circles.

The abstract of Benveniste's paper was as follows:

When humanpolymorphonuclear Basophils, a type of white blood Cell with antibodies of the Immunoglobulin E (Ig E) type on its surface, are exposed to Anti-IgE antibodies, they release histamine from their intracellular granules and change their staining properties. The latter could be demonstrated at dilutions of anti-IgE from 10^2 to 10^{-120}, which naturally implies that most of the experiments with antibody solution re-ported by Benveniste have been carried out in the literal absence of antibody molecules (Figure 4.3).

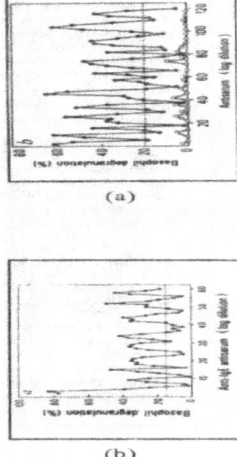

Figure 4.3

Reporting the experiments Benveniste observed that (a) since dilutions need to be accompanied by vigorous shaking for the effects to be observed, transmission of the biological information could be related to the vehicle;

(b) the importance of agitation in the transmission of

information was explored by pipetting dilutions up and down ten times and comparing with the usual 10-second vortexing. Although the two processes resulted in the same dilution, degranulation did not occur at high dilution after simple pipetting ; (c) a striking feature was that molecules reacted to heat according to their distinctive heat sensitivity, whereas all high dilutions ceased to be active between 70°C and 80° C; (d) these results suggested a common mechanism operating at all high dilutions, independent of the nature of the starting molecules; (e) using six biochemical and physical probes, it was confirmed that what supported the activity at high dilutions was not a normal molecule.

Though the Nature's team that visited Benveniste's laboratory did not find the experiments reproducible, the activity was said to be established under stringent experimental condition, such as blind double-coded experiment procedures involving six laboratories from four countries, viz, France, Italy, Canada and Israel.

On 30 June 1088, while publishing the article. Nature's editor observed in an editorial titled "When to believe the unbelievable" that an "article" in that week's issue described observations for which there was no physical basis.

The article showed that it was possible to dilute an aqueous solution of an antibody virtually infinitely without the solution losing its biological activity. The observations were found to be startling not merely because they pointed to a novel phenomenon, but because they struck at the roots of two centuries of observation and rationalization of physical phenomena, such as Law of Mass Action etc.

The chemistry Nobel prize winner Jean-Marie Lahn said in an interview with the French daily 'Lc Monede' — "These results are disturbing, very very disturbing. I do not see how in biology, in the absence of a molecule, information about that molecule can be transmitted."

D. T. Reilly, University of Glasgow, U.K. observed, "Scientific belief belongs on a flat earth. There is no danger, no threat to science in the restatement of the drug diluent paradox. We need only apply the scientific method and then seek the verdict of experience".

K. Opitz, School of Maritime Studies, Hamburg remarked, "Does 'Nature' expect nature to accommodate academic disciplines in order to be vindicated? Casting doubt on findings merely because they are inconvenient to established assumptions and patterns of speculation strikes me as a poor way of advancing scientific knowledge".

Finally it was K. O. Rathhaupt of Max-Planck Institute fur Limnologie, FRG, who commented, "Following the recent correspondences in Nature, I get the impression that there must be something about homoeopathy. I don't believe that no more existent molecules can leave an imprint in water. But isn't it striking how a non-existent phenomenon can leave an imprint in the scientific discussion?"[13]

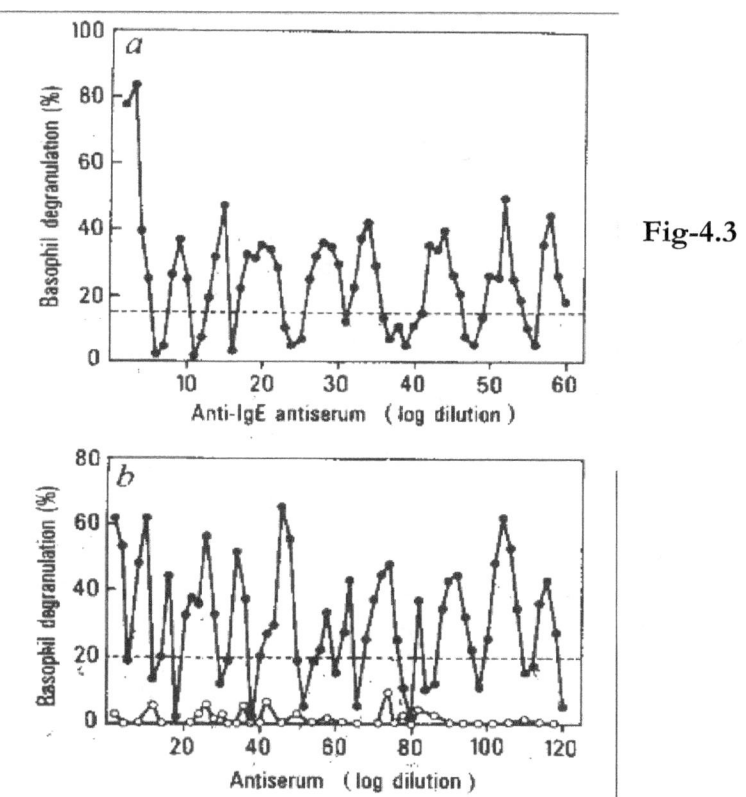

Fig-4.3

5. Concept of Vital Force

As recently as early twentieth century, many scientists were known to be vitalists. They believed that known vital forces operate in living cells, as the mere interaction of their component molecules, according to the familiar laws of science, would not make them live. They observed, therefore, that the fundamental properties of cells such as self-copying inheritance etc, cannot be explained in chemical terms.

In early nineteenth century Berzelius (1815) thought that organic compounds were produced from their elements by laws different from those governing the formation of inorganic compounds. This then led him to believe that organic compounds were produced under the influence of a 'vital force', and that they could not be prepared artificially[14].

Hahnemann (1755-1843), the propounder of the homoeopathic system of treatment, observed that 'the material organism without the vital force s capable of no sensation, function or self preservation. It is thereby dead and subject to the power of the external physical world, it decays and is resolved into its chemical constituents.

It derives all sensation and performs all function of life solely by means of the vital principle, which animates the material organism in health and diseases.'[8] Hahnemann further observed that, 'It is the morbidly affected vital energy alone that produces diseases and the disappearance of all the morbid phenomena, under treatment, necessarily implies the restoration of the integrity of the vital force.' He also believed that the way the vital force caused the organism to display morbid phenomena i.e. produced diseases, would be of no practical utility to the physician to know, neither it would be ever possible for him to know[8].

Justus von Liebig, a great German biochemist of nineteenth century, believed that when the atoms and molecules of a living organism were in their correct relative positions, a new force of nature, the 'vital force', manifested itself in the complex structure of the cell. This force, being inherent in all atoms and molecules, is the principal cause of the molecular reactions and movements at the basis of life and research in biochemistry would therefore reveal the laws of its action, as experiments in physics had revealed the laws of gravitation and electrostatic attraction.

It is true that in 1828 Wohler converted ammonium cyanate into urea, a substance hitherto obtained only from animal sources. But this synthesis had very little effect on the belief in the vital force theory, because it did not start from the elements. Wohler had prepared his ammonium cyanate from ammonia and cyanic acid, both of which were of animal origin. Wohler himself appreciated this point but at that time no methods were known for obtaining ammonia and cyanic acid from their elements. Thus Wohler's synthesis remained incomplete for the time being[14].

It was not until 1845 that the complete synthesis of an organic compound was carried out. In that year Kolbe synthesised acetic acid from its elements. This synthesis was later followed up by others, e.g. in 1856 Berlhelot synthesised methane and thus the concept of vital force got a serious jolt[14].

Notwithstanding that, Hans Driesch, who died in 1940, observed that living organisms differ sharply from non-living in the possession of vital force, which is unlike those familiar to scientists as a purposive directive force. Its purpose being that a living organism should grow' to maturity and reproduce. Resistance of animals to infection was also believed to be one of the characteristics of living organism indicating the existence of this force[15].

Although it is said to be probable that until the brain's activity is fully known the concept of vital force will continue to stay in some form or other, [16] yet spectacular discoveries in molecular biology during the mid-twentieth century undermined the faith of the biologists in vitalism of any kind.

It has been shown that the fundamental properties of living cells, such as their reproducibility and heredity, are founded on the interaction of large molecules i.e. proteins and nucleic acids, according to the normal laws of chemistry. This rendered the concept of vital force, as suggested by Berzelius and others as superfluous[15].

Since long the heredity remained an impenetrable mysticism, in spite of various attempts to explain the same at different times.

Hippocrates, the father of the healing art, propounded the theory that the inherited qualities are transmitted, in some way or other, to the new individual from different parts of the organisms of the parents.

Similar ideas of transmission of qualities from parents to children were also found in the writings of other Greek scientists, inclusive of Aristotle, the great biologist of the olden age.

The last great representative of the transmission theory was, however, Charles Darwin who believed that the cells of the body produced their own miniature copies, called 'gammules', which were carried by the blood into the testes and ovaries, where they were put together to form the gametes. Thus in the new individuals the cells and organs would be replicas of those of the parents. The theory was however, quickly invalidated by his cousin Francis Gallon by blood transfusion experiments on rabbits.

It was only after 1866 when the Augustine monk Gregor Mendel (1822-1884), the father of 'genetics', the science of heredity, published the results of his hybridization experiments on garden peas, the study of heredity was put on firm scientific- basis. Mendel distinguished the essential nature of physical entities and established beyond doubt that heredity consisted of the transmission of these separate units in the reproductive cells, without involving blood or other parts of the body.

Till early twentieth century, however, the concept of 'gene' remained vague and hypothetical. The idea was rather philosophical than tangible reality for experimental research. In about 1910, T.H. Morgan, following his studies on the fruit-fly. Drosophila, first suggested that the chromosomes in the cell nuclei are in reality the carriers of genes, the heredity factors (Figure

5.1 & 5.2).

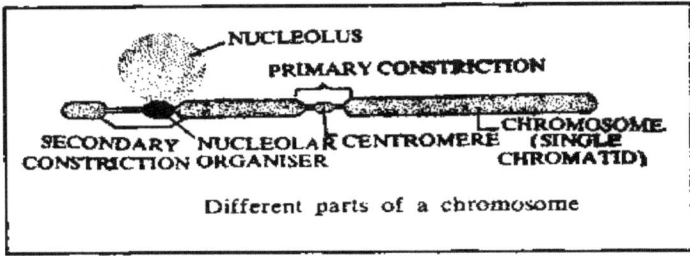

Figure 5.1(a)

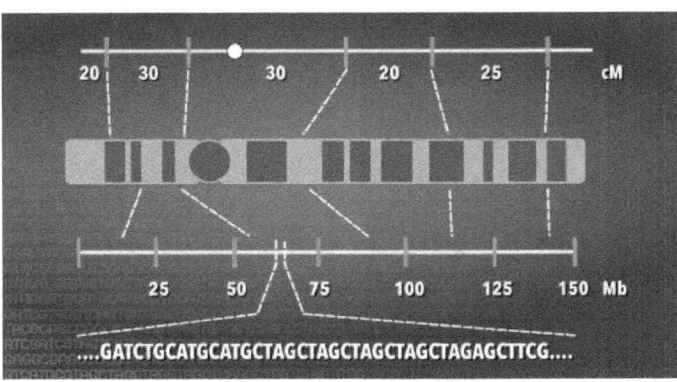

Figure 5.1(b) Genetic Mapping

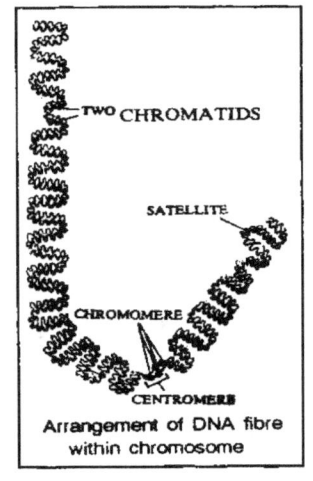

Figure 5.2

Arrangement of DNA fibre within chromosome

In recent years, however, it has been possible to isolate chromosomes from living cells and study extensively their chemical nature and it is now clearly known that chromosomes consist of complex molecules of 'proteins' and 'nucleic acid'.

Proteins and nucleic acid are not only peculiar to living organisms but also inherited differences are said to be linked with the variations of their molecular structure.

Until 1945 proteins were looked on with almost mystical awe by many biochemists am; to suggest their structure took great courage. Today it is known that proteins are built up from a limited number of smaller molecules called amino acids, into which they disintegrate when heated with hydrochloric acid. The molecular weights of proteins are very high, containing some thousands of atoms of carbon, hydrogen, oxygen, nitrogen and sulphur in roughly the same proportion

On the other hand the nucleic acid molecules are also very large and they break down into smaller units called nucleotides, when dissolved in a solution of sodium hydroxide. But whereas a protein molecule contains up to twenty kinds of amino acids, the nucleotides contained in a nucleic acid are normally only of four kinds. Moreover, nucleic acids are of two distinct varieties, ribonucleic acid (RNA) and deoxyribonucleic acid (DNA).

It was originally thought that, the proteins were the

carriers of genetic information but now it is known that such information resides in the molecules of DNA[16].

'Genes' are said to be the segments of DNA molecules that exist in cell nuclei and act by determining synthesis of protein, while the RNA molecules convey the hereditary information to the site of protein production in the cytoplasm and are therefore known as messenger RNA.

It is further known that just as one gene is responsible for the formation of one particular protein, so also one group of nucleotides within the gene is responsible for the insertion of one particular amino acid into the protein.

DNA molecules are known to have helical structures (Figure 5.3). Two strands of alternate sugar

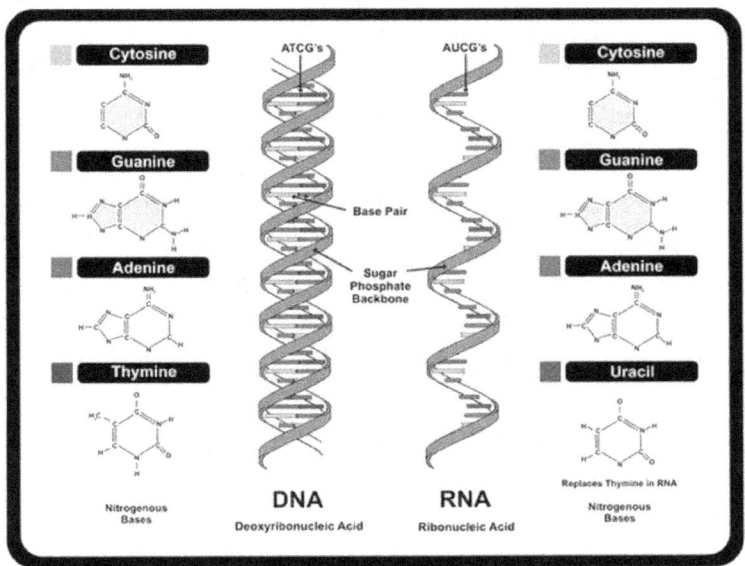

Figure 5.3

(deoxyribose) and phosphate molecules running in opposite directions, with cross links consisting of two bases joined together by weak hydrogen bonds, one strand being wound round another, give a structure antilogous to a spiral staircase.

The sequence of the bases along the molecules is said to specify the individuality with four bases, adenine, cytosine, guanine and thymine. There are 256 (4^4) possible sequences, while in a single molecule consisting tens of thousands of base pairs, the possible sequences would be $4^{10,000}$, each sequence theoretically determining the identity of a different individual. Any change or alteration (mutation) to DNA would be, however, analogous to misprints in the messages arriving at the ribosomes. It was H. J. Muller who in 1927 first discovered the induction of mutation by means of X-Ray radiation (Figure 5.4). Thus while the discoveries of Mendel and Morgan led to better understanding of hereditary diseases, the method of changing the hereditary factors was first found out by Muller.

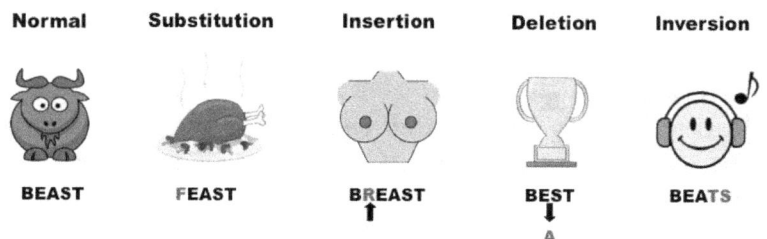

Figure 5.4 (a) Types of Mutation. Each alphabet is a base. Expression of genes change when a base is added, deleted or altered

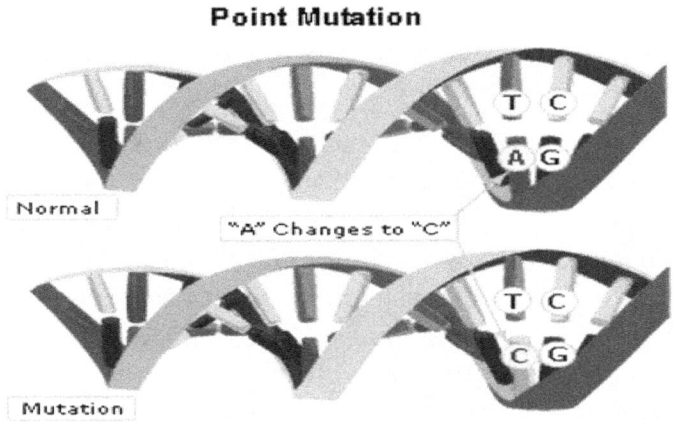

Figure 5.4 (b) Point Mutation

Thus Mendel, Morgan and Muller were not only the three great creators of modern concepts of heredity but also they revolutionized the whole of the biological science.

Today it is known that many of the metabolic disorders, in humans and animals, are due to some defects at the genetic level. While some diseases and illnesses are believed to be genetically determined, there are diseases which are known to be environmentally conditioned. In most of the cases, however, both the factors seem to exists, one of them being predominant over the other[16].

6. Modern Scientific Developments

Throughout the nineteenth century most physicists regarded Newton's dynamical laws as sacrosanct. But it became increasingly clear during the early years of twentieth century that many phenomena, especially those associated with radiation, defy explanation by Newtonian physics.

Although no one had any notion about the way radiation and matter are related or by what process matter emits or absorbs radiation, no one had any doubt that these questions would be answered in time by the proper application of Newton's law of motion and Maxwell's theory of electromagnetic field.

Max Planck's discovery of the quantum of action was an event of first order that changed the whole aspect of physics and deeply influenced all neighboring sciences, from chemistry to biology[17].

Quantum mechanics is concerned with phenomena that are so small-scale that they cannot be described in classical terms, such as may be the ultra-micro doses of potentized homoeopathic medicines.

It is an outgrowth of the concept that all forms of energy are related in discrete units or bundles called 'quanta' and deals with interactions of matter and radiation in terms of observable quantities. Quantum mechanics is in effect an extension of classical statistical mechanics rather than of Newton's deterministic laws.

The quantum field theory is the body of physical principles designed to account for sub-atomic phenomena that also has found application in other branches of physics. The theory arises from attempt to combine the principles of quantum mechanics with those of relativity in an effort to describe processes such as high-energy collisions in which particles may be created or destroyed.

Earlier the notion was that the matter or mass can neither be created nor destroyed. But now it has been observed that natter may be created, for instance by materialization of a quantum of electromagnetic energy (photon or gamma ray) into an electro-positron pair or 'positronium'. Also matter may be destroyed by annihilation of this pair of elementary particles to pair of gamma rays[18].

Further, until 1900, physicists believed that matter and energy were two distinct realms in nature governed by different laws. Pure energy, manifesting itself as radiation, was thought of entirely in terms of 'waves', whereas matter was considered to be entirely 'corpuscular' in nature. Today the existence of corpuscle accompanied by wave properties are known to be assumed in all cases, both matter and energy.

The wave and the particle pictures are said to be complementary aspects of the same physical entity and one must exist at the expense of the other (Figure 6.1).

The 'electron' has this diffused wave character so long as we do not try to observe it, for as soon as we look for it and find it as a particle, we immediately condense it into a small wave packet, concentrated in a small region of space.

The more accurately we observe its position, the less diffused its wave-like character becomes and the more do its corpuscular properties manifest themselves[18].

Further, Schwinger's electro-dynamics suggests that a free electron is accompanied by an electromagnetic field, which effectively alters the inertia of the system and an electromagnetic field is accompanied by a current of electron-positron pairs, i.e. positronium, which effectively alters the strength of the field and all charges[18].

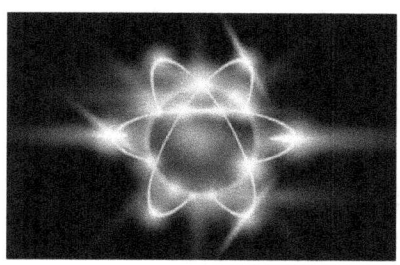 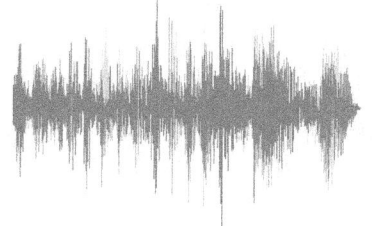

Figure 6.1

(a) Particle (b) Wave

The chemical properties of atom is, however known to be determined by the electronic configuration i.e. the mode of arrangement and the number of electrons required to make the atom neutral.

To elaborate it may be mentioned that molecules (Figures 6.2) are the units of matter, the smallest portion of an element or compound that retains chemical identity with the substance in mass. It consists of a group of atoms, ranging from

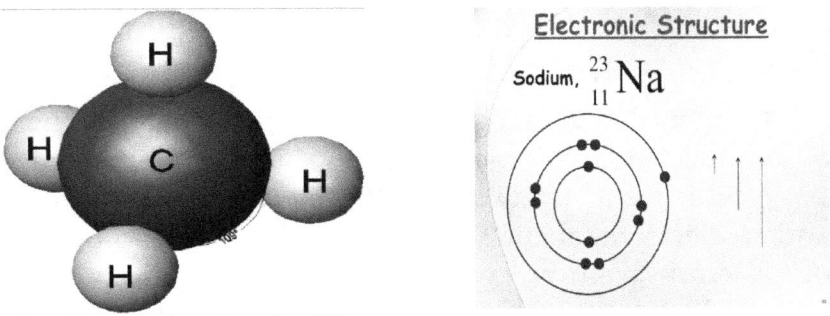

Figure 6.2

(a) Molecule   (b) Atom

One in inert gases to very large numbers in organic chain molecules. Atoms are however, largely empty, consisting of a small solid core, the 'nucleus', which is surrounded by a number of negatively charged particles called 'electrons'.

The electrons circulate around the nucleus in separate orbits, while nucleus is a composite structure consisting of several sub-units, 'protons' and 'neutrons' held firmly together. The simplified picture of the atom" (Figure 6.3), therefore, involves three particles, the 'neutron' with unit mass and zero charge, 'proton' with unit mass and unit positive charge and the 'electron' with infinitely small mass and unit negative charge. Neutrons and protons are again believed to be formed of the hypothetical basic particles 'Quarks'. So 'electrons' and 'quarks' are the two elementary particles so far known.

Number of electrons present in an atom is known to be its 'atomic number', which is independent of the mass of the atom i.e. atomic weight.

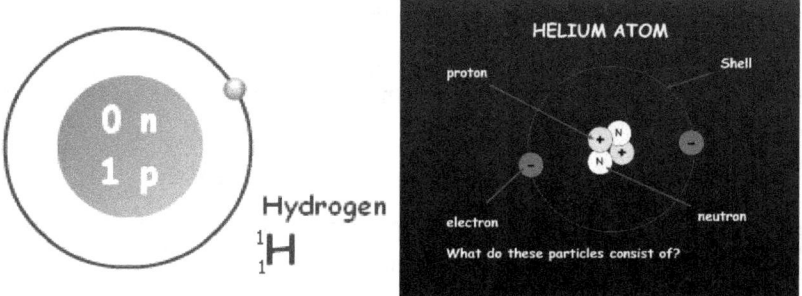

Figure 6.3
(a) Hydrogen (b) Helium atoms

Atoms of the same element having same atomic number but different atomic weights are known as 'isotopes' of the element. Isotopes are identical in chemical behaviour and distinguishable by small difference in their atomic weights only. This is due to their having same number of protons but different number of neutrons in the nucleus (Figure 6.4). Many of the common elements are known to be mixtures of their isotopes.

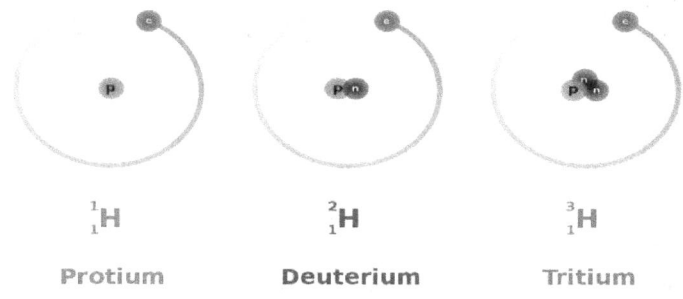

Figure 6.4*(hydrogen is also known as 'protium', i.e. electron – proton pair)*

Similarly, molecules having the same chemical constitution and structure but differing in that—one or more atoms in one are isotopically different from the corresponding atoms in the other are said to be 'isotopic molecules'.

'Positron' (the positive electron) is the unit of elementary positive charge having the same mass, spin, magnitude of charge and magnetic moment as that of electron. Positron is extremely unstable in the presence of electron. It is comparatively rare particle and is observed principally in cosmic radiation and also in the emission of some artificial radioactive (unstable) isotopes. In the vicinity of an electron, a positron is known to be annihilated, giving rise to one or more quanta of gamma radiation, with a characteristic total energy of 1.0216 MeV, the sum of the rest masses of the two particles

Certain characteristic of the process is how-ever influenced if the particles meet in an atomic environment. In many cases, especially in gases, the annihilation takes place not in a free collision but after formation of an intermediary system called 'positronium', where the electron and the positron are bound to each other (e^+ e^-) by the electromagnetic force.

Formation of positronium is also known to be promoted by application of an electric field. It is known that when an electron comes somewhere near the nucleus of an atom, where there are strong electric fields, the electron is accelerated and in the course of that it gives of a gamma ray and then the electron goes on with a little less energy. Then if the gamma ray comes near the nucleus of another atom it makes a pair, an electron-positron (e^+ e^-) pair.

Gamma rays are known as electromagnetic waves, similar to visible light but with very short wave lengths and no change in atomic number or atomic weight is said to be caused by emission of gamma rays.

The pair production is of considerable theoretical interest in particle science, not only as an example of materialization of energy, but also as a striking confirmation of the relativistic quantum theory proposed by Dirac.

The existence of positronium, an electron-positron atomic system of infinitely small mass, has however been established through indirect evidences, as observation became difficult due to considerable Doppler broadening caused by the relatively high velocity of atoms of such small mass at thermal energies[19].

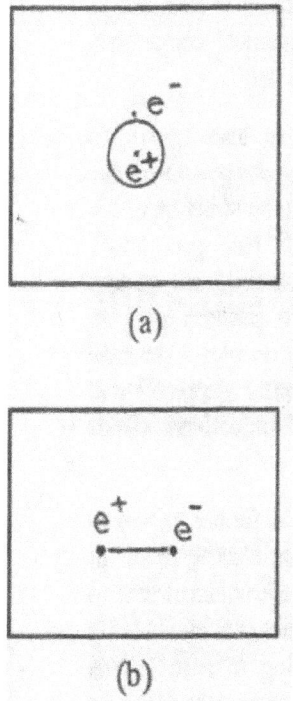

Figure 6.5
Light isotope of hydrogen
(a) Positronium or
b) Electron-positron pair.

Further, positronium is structurally analogous to a hydrogen atom. The gross structure of its energy levels being same as that of hydrogen the fine structure is rather different. In hydrogen atom one electron revolves about a single proton, whereas in positronium the part of the proton is played by a positron. Hence positronium is said to behave like a very light isotope of hydrogen.[20]. (Figure 6.5.)

Apart from its short life (10^{-7} to 10^{-10} second) the mass and charge centres in the alliance are known to be coincident. During its brief lifetime positronium is also said to be capable of entering into chemical compounds which have free valance bonds left[21].

Stability of positronium is also known to depend markedly on the chemical composition of the surrounding medium and also on the structure of the molecules the electron-positron pair gets into[22]. Existence of positronium complexes, such as two electrons plus a positron, two positron plus an electron, an electron plus a positron and like that have been theoretically accepted[22] and in some cases formation of positronium compounds have also been suggested[19].

Formation of positronium is further known to be promoted by application of an electric field. In some gases the production of positronium is said to be enhanced to almost hundred per cent by applying electric fields[23]. It is interesting to note in this context the observation of J. Maddox, the Nature's editor that - 'Electron-positron pairs can be created out of nothing, anywhere and anytime by the so called fluctuation of vacuum of the electromagnetic fields[24].'

Beside positronium, the light isotope of 'hydrogen', existence of two more such light isotopes, e.g. the light isotope of 'helium' and light isotope of 'lithium', (Figure 6.6) have also been confirmed in recent time[25].

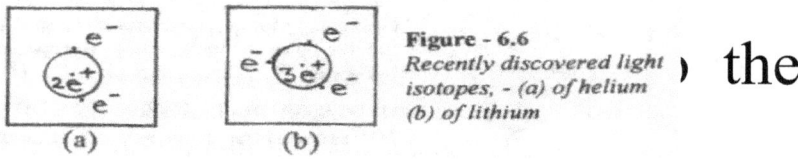

Figure - 6.6
Recently discovered light isotopes, - (a) of helium (b) of lithium

In the process of homoeopathic potentization the very first thing that occurs is the production of electromagnetic fields, due to friction between ethanol molecules and the glass surface.

Individual atoms or large group of atoms and molecules of many substances are known to have an affinity for additional electrons. Electron affinity, the characteristic of non-metal, is, however, said to be dependent upon the size of the atom. Therefore, the affinity for more electrons varies from atom to atom and when two different substances are brought into contact, the substance with greater affinity for electrons seizes nearby electrons from the atom of the other substance.

The elementary character of the atom however does not change due to excess or deficiency of electron, as because this is known to depend on the protons existing in the nucleus of the atom, which cannot be easily separated.

A substance thus having on its surface more electrons than protons is said to be negatively charged, while the one having more protons than electrons is positively charged. Thus electrostatic charge or static electricity is found to develop in many non-metallic substances such as glass, resins, plastics etc. The excess type of charge commonly associated with resins was however originally termed as 'resinous electricity' and deficiency type characteristic of glass was called 'vitreous electricity'. A piece of amber (natural resin) as big as the end segment of a man's finger is known to acquire and hold as many as 100,000,000 (hundred millions) excess electrons in less than a second.

As rubbing or friction further increases the charge due to intensive contact between the surfaces of the two bodies, it is also known as 'frictional electricity'. As continued friction causes addition of more and more electrons to a substance, separated from another substance, so in the process high voltage can be developed due to high potential differences. Static electricity is thus said to be of high voltage although of low-current type.

Not only an insulating or insulated solid body acquires frictional electricity by rubbing it with other bodies, whether insulating or conducting, but also charges are known to be generated when a liquid flows over a solid surface[26], one or both of which may be an insulator. Large charges are also known to be produced by blowing powders against a solid surface[26]. Only good insulators are, however, known to show a net charge after rubbing, because electric conduction permits neutralization of the charges very rapidly in other materials.

The homoeopathic process of potentization or dynamization consists of serial dilution followed by succussion, or trituration. During succussion or trituration, either the ethanol molecules are vigorously flown over the inner surface of the glass vials or the lactose powder is strongly rubbed against the inner wall of the porcelain mortar with the pestle, thereby causing development of electric field.

As in the case of succussion, at every stage new glass vial and fresh ethanol are taken, the process becomes open and continuous. But in case of trituration the same mortar and pestle is used all along, so after some time the process of generation of electric field may become stagnated.

Alcohol due to stronger electron affinity acquires excess electrons and gets negatively charged while the glass surface due to deficiency in electron becomes positively charged. The charges so developed are however not easily neutralized by conduction, because the glasses, especially the commercial glasses used, are known to be highly resistive to electricity, which is known to be extremely high, particularly in room temperature. Velvet cork, porcelain mortar-pestles, ebonite spatula etc. are also known to be highly resistive to electricity. It is to be particularly noted in this context that the medicinal value of the homoeopathic potencies are said to be not developed if touched by hand during the process of preparation. This is so because the charges thus produced are easily conducted through body.

Thus in the process of homoeopathic potentization increasingly strong electric fields are produced. Incidentally it may be noted here that the glass vessels, particularly of straight cylindrical types, are known to be capable of withstanding very high voltage [27].

In the strong electric fields thus produced, as observed earlier, it may be conceived that through absorption of electro-magnetic waves electron-positron pairs or positronium units are created (Figure 7.1).

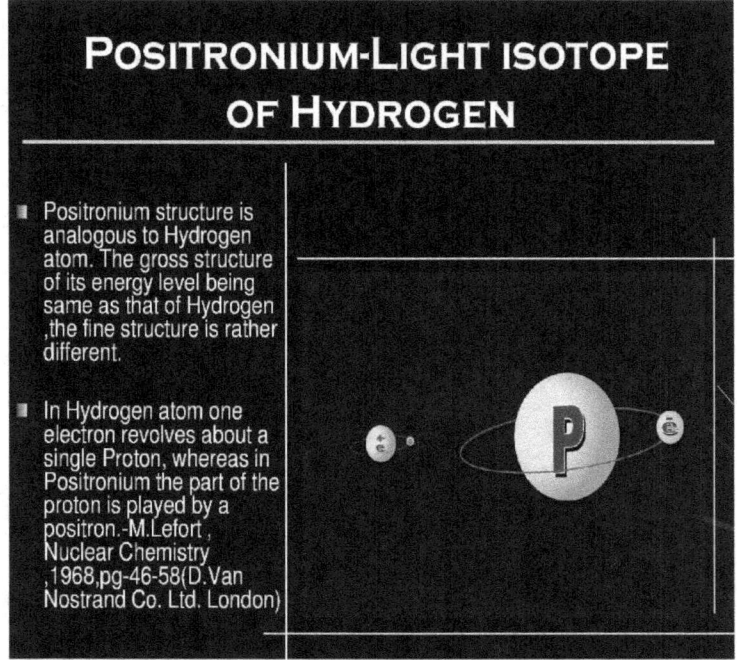

POSITRONIUM-LIGHT ISOTOPE OF HYDROGEN

- Positronium structure is analogous to Hydrogen atom. The gross structure of its energy level being same as that of Hydrogen, the fine structure is rather different.

- In Hydrogen atom one electron revolves about a single Proton, whereas in Positronium the part of the proton is played by a positron.-M.Lefort, Nuclear Chemistry ,1968,pg-46-58(D.Van Nostrand Co. Ltd. London)

Homoeopathy in the Light of Modern Science

SOME FACTS ABOUT POSITRONIUM

- During brief life time Positronium is also said to be capable of entering into chemical compounds which have free valence bonds left.- Vlasov. L. Trifonov.D, 107 stories about Chemistry, 1972(Mir publishers,Moscow)pg.210-212

- Stability of Positronium is further known to depend markedly on the Chemical composition of the surrounding medium and also on the structure of the molecules , the electron positron pair gets into-Heissnisky M., Nuclear Chemistry and its application,1964(Addison-Weley pub. U.S.A.)pg 33-34.

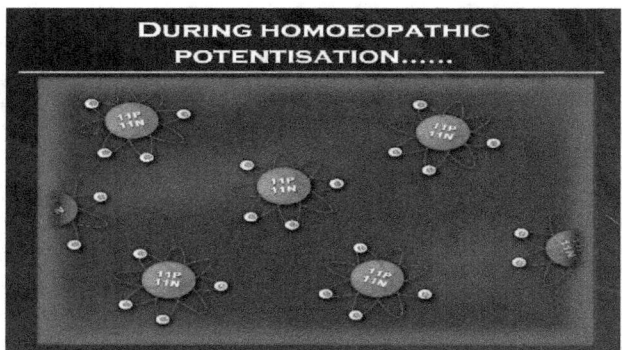

During homoeopathic potentisation......

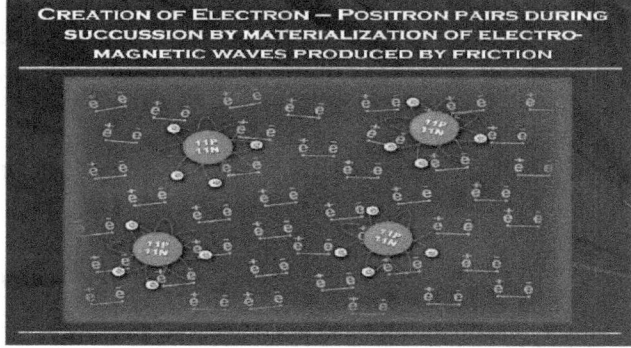

Creation of Electron – Positron pairs during succussion by materialization of electro-magnetic waves produced by friction

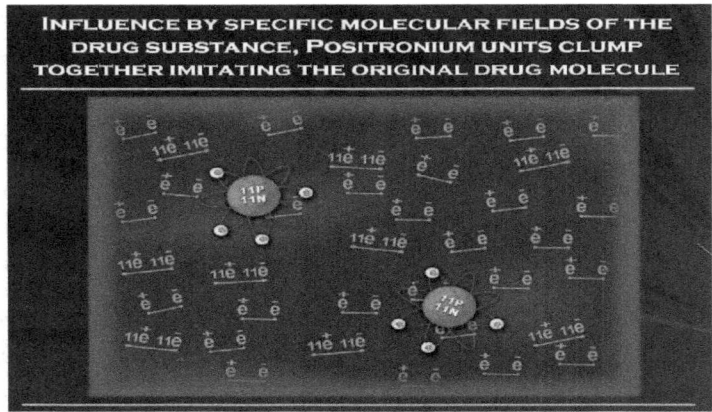

INFLUENCE BY SPECIFIC MOLECULAR FIELDS OF THE DRUG SUBSTANCE, POSITRONIUM UNITS CLUMP TOGETHER IMITATING THE ORIGINAL DRUG MOLECULE

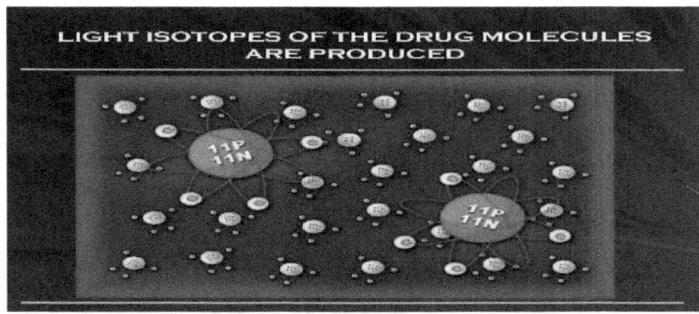

LIGHT ISOTOPES OF THE DRUG MOLECULES ARE PRODUCED

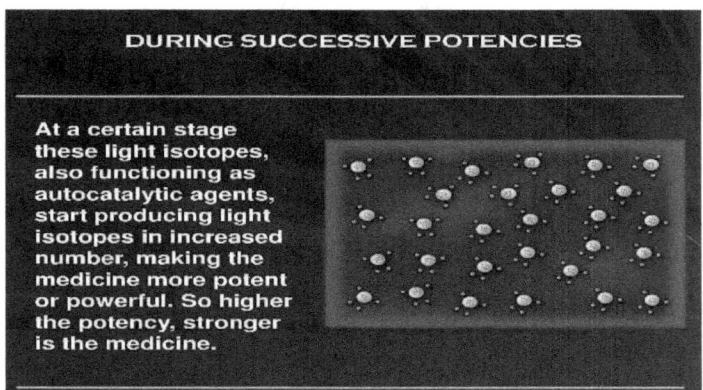

DURING SUCCESSIVE POTENCIES

At a certain stage these light isotopes, also functioning as autocatalytic agents, start producing light isotopes in increased number, making the medicine more potent or powerful. So higher the potency, stronger is the medicine.

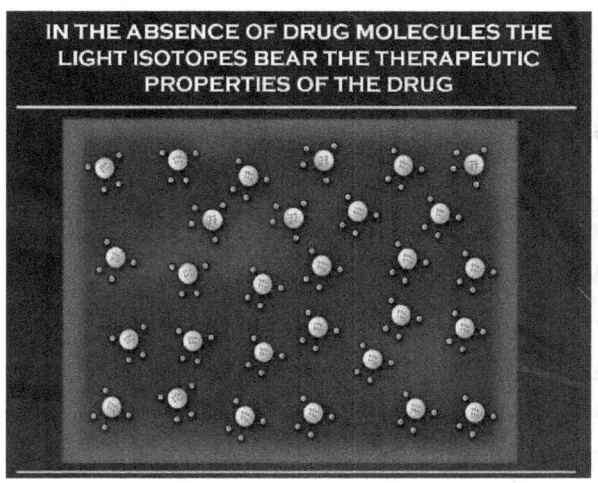
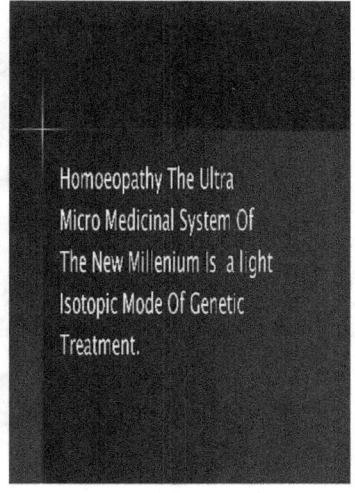

Fig 7.1

The positronium units thus created in the surroundings of the polar molecules of ethanol are not only supposed to be more stable but also expected to clump together to give rise to various positronium complexes, with or without interaction with 'neutrinos', the baby neutrons.

The creation of neutrino is known to require negligible energy, since its rest mass is close to zero.

Further, the polarity has been recognized as an important factor in determining the effects of specific interactions and orientation of the different kinds of molecules. Polar solvents are not only known to induce moments in non-polar solute molecules, but also such polar molecules, if placed in an electric field, are expected to become oriented in that field just as a bar of magnet placed in a magnetic field becomes aligned with the magnetic field[28].

According to some recent observations, micro-scopic particles in suitable environment are known to behave like mini-magnets. The properties of such mini-magnets, their strength and orientation and ability to change either, are also said to depend crucially on the characteristics of the host, in the vicinity of the atom or ion[29].

Thus it may be postulated that in the vicinity of the drug molecules and induced by their specific molecular fields, some of the positronium units will clump together specifically so as to imitate the electronic arrangement of the drug molecules. Such positronium complexes formed, are then expected to behave like very light isotope of the original drug molecules and retain their therapeutic properties even in their absence[13]. Specific clumping of some positronium units imitating the electronic configuration of carbon atoms.

Further, it may also be postulated that at certain stage these light isotopic molecules functioning as auto-catalytic agent will continue to give rise to their next generations in proportionately increasing concentrations, thereby making the homoeopathic potencies more and more powerful with higher degree of dynamization[13].

Mathematical expression for an 'auto-catalytic' action is, however, known to require that no catalyst is present in the beginning of the reaction and the reaction velocity is proportional to the concentration of the reaction product[30].

A theoretical substantiation for the above postulation is also found in the following recent observation: 'A curiosity is that nature seems to be making Xerox copies of the basic pattern shown by the up and down quarks, together with the electronic neutrino and electron. These Xerox copies seem to differ just in their mass and copy number. The copy number is also referred to as generation[31].

A peculiar 'off' and 'on' effect with the homoeopathic potencies giving a curve of sinusoidal type, as observed by Nebel, Boyd, Benveniste and others, can only be ascribed to an auto-catalytic effect generated in the process of potentization.

For any auto-catalytic reaction proceeding in a liquid phase, the velocity of the reaction is said to gradually increase with the increase in the concentration of the catalyst. But when a decrease in the concentration of the reactants, counteract this influence of the concentration of the catalyst, the velocity of the reaction is decreased. Auto-catalytic reactions are therefore graphically expressed by the curve of sine-type[30].

Substances such as common salt, sand, alumina etc. having practically no medicinal value in their crude forms, are known to develop some kind of toxicity in the process of potentization and thereby achieving extraordinary medicinal power, in their homoeopathic potencies. This may be ascribed only to their light isotopic forms. Because isotopes, though having similar chemical properties, are often known to act biochemically at different rates due to their differences in activation energy. Thus water, possessing no toxic effect for any life process, its isotopic form 'heavy water' is a retarder up to a poison.

Further, homoeopathic potentized medicines are known to be less heat stable. This is because the structure of substances on the molecular scale is known to be determined by a balance between the ordering influence of intermolecular forces and the disordering influence of thermal motion.

In the homoeopathic potencies as postulated above, the positronium units are supposed to be specifically clumped together by comparatively weak electromagnetic force. Hence they are naturally less heat stable, although the original drug molecules may differently react to heat according to their distinctive heat sensitivity.

Incidentally the wooden chest, glass vessels, velvet cork and paper packs generally used for preserving potentized homoeopathic medicines are all known as highly resistive to heat. A dose of potentized homoeopathic remedy in its paper envelope in the desk is said to retain its medicinal virtue for years. Homoeopathic potencies are also advised to be kept protected from sunlight and even external body heat.

Potentized homoeopathic medicines due to their light isotopic forms are also expected to be capable of penetrating into the chromosome level and exert their corrective influences on the defective genes, without themselves being observable.

In the globular doses of increasingly higher

homoeopathic potencies there is increasing concentration of high energy light isotopic molecules. In other words a single globular dose of the same homoeopathic medicine in 6c, 12c, 30c. 200c or 1000c or 100,000c potencies arc atomistic and therefore increasingly quantized and discontinuous[17].

The importance of quantum of action for life process is indicated by the continuity and remarkable stability of the genes. The genes can only change their structure discontinuous and not gradually. If action were not quantized even small environmental changes would change the genetic structure[17].

Thus the 'light isotopic model' of homoeopathic potentized medicine[13] is not only based on modern scientific concepts and capable of resolving the potency phenomena most satisfactorily but also for the first time in remaining fully consistent with the law of mass action, surpasses the Avogadrian impasse, the historical stumbling block against any scientific acceptance of homoeopathic system of medicine.

8. Modus Operandi

Almost since its inception the homoeopathic system of medicine was under continuous challenge. All attempts made to establish it in corroboration with modern scientific concepts remained either inadequate or totally unacceptable.

Large number of cures, some verging even to miraculous, hardly received any appreciation from the scientific circles and the claims of cure were simply attributed to either psychological or natural phenomena.

In the beginning administration of insignificantly small homoeopathic doses and claims of cure thereby was just a matter of ridicule to many. This became all the more apparent when in late nineteenth century Louis Pasteur and Robert Koch established beyond any doubt the 'germ theory', and it was found that potentized homoeopathic remedies do not possess any direct deadly effect on the specific disease producing germs.

Further, with the resurrection of Avogadro's number on the one hand and on the other hand the concept of vital force becoming obsolete, the curative power as well as the mode of action of homoeopathic potentized medicines remained scientifically inconceivable. But when viewed from a genetic standpoint, the scientific basis of the micro- medicinal system seems to unveil itself, that baffled the scientific community for nearly two hundred years.

Today it is known that mere implantation of micro-organism on the surface membrane, e.g. skin, mucosae, conjunctiva etc. accompanied by its reproduction is not sufficient to constitute disease.

In a susceptible person in whom the natural defense mechanism of the body is defective, the organism establishes itself in the tissues, multiply freely, produce its toxic substances and give rise to a typical attack of the disease, while in an immune person the infection may be completely resisted and the organism destroyed before any damage is done.

In homoeopathy, therefore, protection against the toxin produced by a bacterium is more important than against the micro-organism itself, since the symptoms of the disease are primarily due to the toxin and not the presence of the bacteria in the body. The size of the bacteria is not apparently injurious and they do not multiply to such an extent that may interfere with the activities of the body by shear bulk[33].

During the progress of an infection, acquired immunity develops and antibodies are produced in certain cells of the body which act on the particular type of micro-organism responsible for infection.

It is interesting to note that many of the recent researches in the fields of immunotherapy, vaccinotherapy, allergy etc. show surprising similarity with that of homoeopathic system of treatment.

Hahnemann observed, "Every artificial morbific agent acts upon the vitality to cause certain alteration in the health of the individual to which the vital force rouses itself to develop the exact opposite condition of health[8]". This appears strikingly analogous to the recent finding that there is a long list of offending substances known as allergen, capable of producing an altered reaction in an animal, to which the body immediately reacts to protect itself[34].

The chemical substances that trigger the reaction in the body are known as 'antigen' and the chemical substances produced by the body to combat and neutralize such antigens are known as 'antibodies'. The union between the antibody and the corresponding substance in the micro-organism referred to as antigen is highly specific, resembling a lock-and-key mechanism.

The homoeopathic remedies are also known as highly symptom specific. In each case of disease, there is the specific homoeopathic remedy, which is found to contain in the symptoms, the greatest similarity to the totality of symptoms of a given natural disease.

The uncommonly minute dose of homoeopathic medicine is also comparable to the amount of antigen needed to sensitize an animal, which is remarkably small, the limit being of the order of one ten- thousandth of a milligram.

Desensitizing method to combat allergies by exposing the allergic patient to small quantities of the antigen in increasing doses is also comparable to the use of accurately chosen homoeopathic remedies in properly small and gradually increasing doses, to avoid undesired aggravation.

For identification of an allergen, the detailed history of the condition, its evolution, exact location in the body, when it improves, the effect of the seasons etc. are necessarily obtained through questioning the patient, which is similar to that of homoeopathic system of treatment.

The degree of immunity resulting from the administration of a vaccine is also known to be variable, depending on the potency of antigen preparation, the doses given, the interval between doses and the degree of ability (sensitivity) of the person to produce antibodies, when properly stimulated[32]. All these remind one of the homoeopathic system of treatment.

However, homoeopathic drug substances are not always necessarily 'proteins' as in case of antigens. But it is important to note in this context that as per recent observations, substances other than protein may form loose complexes with the protein of the body and the complexes may serve as antigens and stimulate the production of 'reagin', the hypothetical antibody[33].

Therefore, it may not be a matter of wonder to guess that the light isotopic molecules (positronium complexes) formed in the higher homoeopathic potencies, where the original drug molecules no longer exist, form loose complexes with the protein of the body and trigger a highly specific antigen- antibody-like reaction.

The immune response to various 'antigens' is, however, known to be under the controlling influence of genes, termed as immune response (Ir) genes. The genes are present in all vertebrates including man, where they may influence the outcome of various diseases.

Today it is known that many of the metabolic

disorders in humans and animals are due to some defects in the genetic level. Although generally quite stable, a gene subjected to unusual stress may undergo a sudden permanent change known as gene mutation. Normally mutations are known to bring forth basic biochemical changes and are harmful to organism.

In addition to ionizing radiation and ultra-violet rays, many chemical compounds have been found to be mutagenic. A recent finding that the coli bacteria can be responsible for more than doubling the spontaneous mutation frequency has upset many old notions including the traditional distinction between heredity and infection[34].

By some recent experiment with bacteriophages, bacteria, neurospora and silkworms, it has been observed that genes mutate at different relative frequencies on treatment with different chemical agents. This is indicative of the possibility that mutation process may be directed by suitable chemicals capable of inducing particular mutation[35].

Back or 'Reverse Mutation' from a mutant to its normal type allele is also known to occur[35], and utilizing forward and reverse mutations induced by some chemicals a model of molecular mutagenesis has already been proposed in bacteriophages by Freese[36]. In higher organisms, however, such a precise study with these mutagens is said to be difficult in view of the complex nature of the genetic and chromosomal organization .

Further, it has been observed that mutation in fungus Neurospora, resulting in changes in DNA molecules, led to mutant strains deficient in enzymes necessary for 'arginin' synthesis. But by addition of 'streptomycin' to the growth medium, some of these mutations could be corrected, thereby enabling the mutant strains to synthesize Arginine. This was believed to have profound implications, because if the same was found to be true of human DNA, it might be possible to correct mutation in man by means of some chemical agencies.

According to some recent observations, gene mutations, although not yet fully understood, are believed to be caused by some ultramicroscopic events of molecular or sub molecular motions[33], and any agent that can penetrate to the chromosomes, having a localized chemical effect, can exert its influences into the genetic information, provided the cells are not killed earlier by other mechanisms[32].

The genetic information in all living cells is encoded in DNA molecules, and it was earlier believed that information is sequentially transferred from DNA to RN A to protein. But with the discovery of a viral enzyme called 'reverse transcriptage', the reverse flow of genetic information from protein to nucleic acid has been confirmed[37].

Discovery of 'prostaglandins' in body fluids and tissues, its specific effects and its production and release evoked by stimulation of nerves, indicate the meeting ground of two main systems of communication in the body, 'hormones' and the 'nerves', meeting directly in the membrane of the cell[38]. Varieties of environmental signals are again believed to be received and transferred by cell surface receptors. (Figure-8.1 & 8.2)

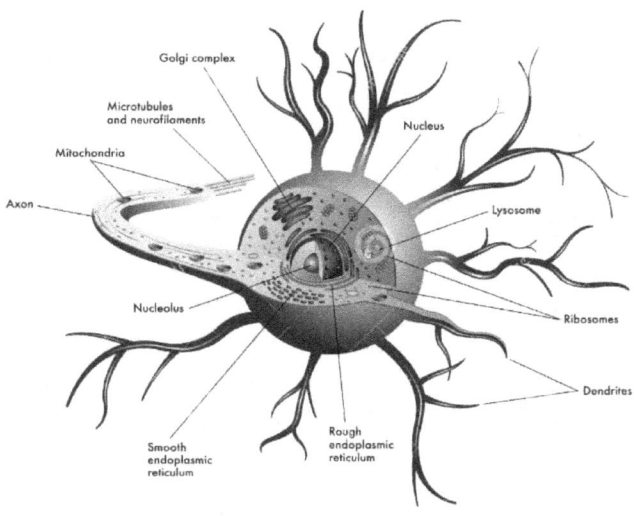

Figure 8.1

Neuron (nerve cell)

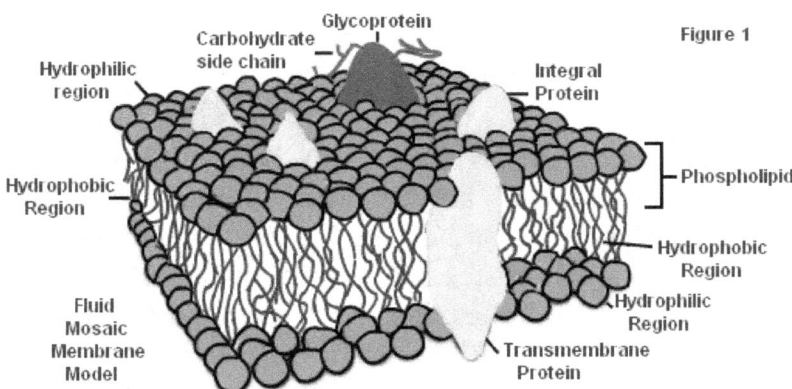

Figure 8.2

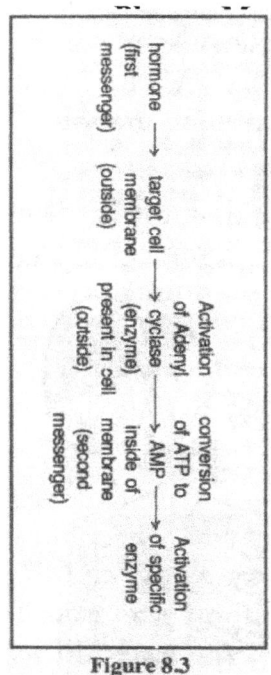
...nbrane (A living ultra-thin covering of ...sm of plant and animal cells)

Figure 8.3
Hormones
(Its mechanism of action)

The binding of such a signaling legend or 'First Messenger' induce a change in the receptor, initiating the next events by which information is carried across the membranes into the cell interior. The cyclic nucleotides, cyclic AMP(Adenosine monophosphate) and cyclic GMP(Guanosine monophosphate), which are regulated by specific membrane bound enzymes (cyclases), have received much attention as a 'Second Messenger' in the signaling cellular activity[39]. (Figure - 8.3)

Due to extraordinary minute-ness of the dose, the homoeopathic medicine is believed to be transient and disappears rapidly of its own. The original 'antigen' introduced in the body is also known to be eliminated quickly during the process of renewal of the whole structure of an animal, while the stamp set by a course of immunization remains and the synthesis of antibody or at least a heightened capacity to form antibody persists without fresh introduction of antigen. This is due to the fact that the human plasma cells make considerable amount of RNA and possibly the cell reads the same RNA blue-prints over and over in its manufacture of the antibody[15].

In the process of homoeopathic treatment it has been observed that diseases of long standing, and especially such as are of complicated character, require for their cure a proportionately long time, while recently developed acute diseases disappear imperceptibly in few hours under the action of proper homoeopathic remedies.

Moreover, in chronic cases, disease symptoms are known to get well in the reverse order of their coming. The last symptoms will be the first to go away, and that the older symptoms will come and go in reverse order in which they appeared. Where the old symptoms do not come back the disease process is said to be restrained and not cured.

Hence it may be inferred that the homoeopathic potentized medicines, due to their light-isotopic forms, are capable of penetrating into the chromosome level and exert their chemical influences for the correction of genetic defects.

Thus in acute cases, functioning like 'antigens', they artificially stimulate the body's antigen-anti- body-like immunological responses, in specific direction, thereby promptly curing the diseases. (Figure- 8.4) Whereas in chronic diseases, functioning like 'mutagens', they trigger the body's specific "Reverse Mutation" (Figure 8.5) processes, when the disease symptoms reappear in the reverse order of their coming, until the disease is fully cured.

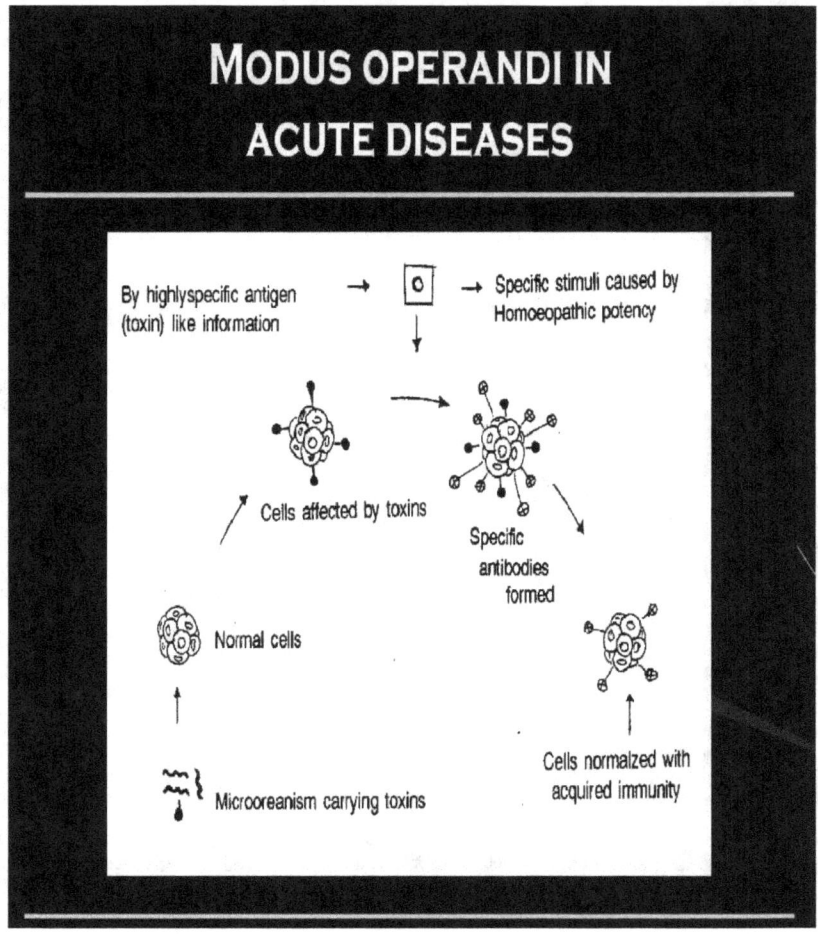

Figure 8.4: *Action of homeopathic potentized medicines in acute diseases.*

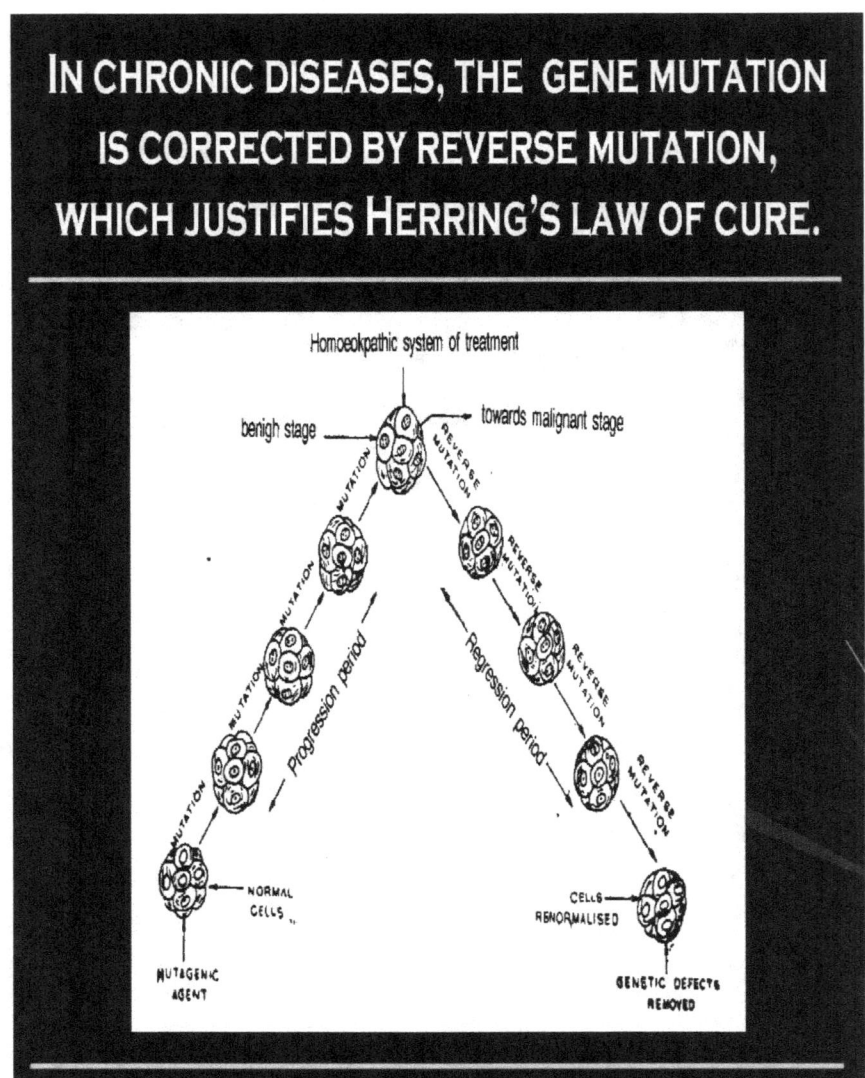

Figure 8.5:*Action of homoeopathic potencies in chronic diseases.*

9. Chronic Miasm

According to conventional thinking a disease that runs for less than six weeks is known to be acute and if it runs for an indefinite period, it is termed as chronic. In homoeopathy however, a disease is characterized acute or chronic, from the very beginning, depending on as nature and the inherent Miasm in it[9].

During his long experience, Hahnemann observed that chronic diseases of non-venereal origin always returned in a more or less varied form and with new symptoms or reappeared annually with an increase of complaints and also that after it had once advanced and developed to a certain degree, it could never be removed by the strength of most robust constitution, the best regulated mode of living, nor will it die out of itself. Even the new additions of proved medicines, increasing from year to year, did not advance the healing of these diseases by a single step, while acute diseases were speedily and completely cured by means of correct application of homoeopathic remedies.

Hahnemann further observed that most of the non-venereal chronic diseases were found to originate from an acknowledged preceding itch, when that had not been cured from within. This led Hahnemann to conclude that the chronic maladies, when they are not of syphilitic or sycotic origin, spring from the Miasm (noxious influence) of itch.

According to Hahnemann, therefore, all chronic diseases of mankind must have for their origin and foundation, constant chronic miasms, whereby their parasitical existence in the human organism is enabled to continually rise and grow, To be more precise, the three chronic miasms, 'psora' (internal itch malady), 'sycosis' (figwart disease) and 'syphilis' (venereal chancre disease) are responsible for most, if not all the chronic diseases, which manifest themselves through local symptoms.

This further led Hahnemann to the discovery of a series of deep acting remedies, far more specific for chronic affections arising from psora, sycosis, syphilis and were termed as 'anti-psoric', 'anti-sycotic' and 'anti-syphilitic' remedies.

Further, all the three chronic miasms were said to be contagious in nature, of which psora was the oldest, most common and most contagious. It had been further observed that the infection with miasms of the acute as well as the chronic diseases take place without doubt in one single moment and that moment is the one most favourable for infection.

In this connection one very important observation made by Hahnemann was found to be broadly true and accepted afterwards by the medical world. He observed, "With respect to the origin of these chronic maladies, as in acute miasmatic eruptional disease, three different important moments are to be considered more attentively than has hitherto been done. First, the time of infection; secondly, the period of time during which the whole organism is being penetrated by the disease infused, until it has developed within; and thirdly, the breaking out of the external ailment, whereby nature externally demonstrates the completion of the internal development of this miasmatic malady throughout the whole organism[9].

It is, however, known that the 'incubation period', elapsing between the access of the infecting organism to the body and the appearance of manifested symptoms of a disease varies greatly. At one end of the scale is acute streptococcal septicaemia which may be fatal within 24 hours and at the other end is a disease such as leprosy, caused by bacillus Mycobacterium leprae, where infection may be beyond clinical evidence for years.

Literally 'psora' means itching disease of the skin, more specifically scabies or itch, and psoriasis. While scabies or itch, caused by a species of mite. 'Sarcoptes scabiei'. is known to be highly contagious and the disease is characterized by intense itching, especially at night, with rash, follicular papules or vesicles, there is no evidence on the other hand that the psoriasis is in the least contagious and so far no infectious agent has been isolated from the lesions of psoriasis.

Some other contagious skin diseases are also known to be caused by certain fungal bacterial or viral infection, such as ringworm, impetigo, warts, molluscum contagiosum etc. Broadly speaking, the human skin is subject to a large number of diseases, some of them inconsequential, others chronic and productive of prolonged partial or total disability and the rest associated with internal medical diseases of varying seriousness.

Miasmatically also 'psora' and itch are not identical.

While psora is said to be a condition of a man, a condition that favours diseases, itch is merely an indication of existence of psora[40].

So also, 'sycosis' is not gonorrhoea but it is said to be the condition of human system, that is bonded to it by gonorrhoea, which was not cured but only made to disappear either by a course of suppressive treatment or by itself. Similarly, syphilis' is a condition of the system arising out of the suppression of the chancre[40].

Literally, however, 'sycosis' has been derived from the word 'sykon' meaning fig. Hahnemann has however, also called sycosis as the 'condylomatous disease' or the figwart miasm. It may be noted in this context that the venereal warts are known to be caused by certain virus infection. Similarly, syphilis has also been called by him as venereal chancre miasm.

By 1910 the causative organism of syphilis was definitely known as Spirochaete Treponema Pallidum. The incubation period of the organism varies from 10 to 90 days, with an average of about 21 days. The primary lesion is characterized by a chancre and regional buboes. The chancre being a tissue reaction at the portal of entry of the organism, composed of granulation tissue which forms a hardened ulcer. If left untreated, a series of recurring lesions of the skin or mucosa may occur during the first two years. From 3 to 30 or even more years after infection, a late or tertiary manifestation may occur which might kill, incapacitate, or affect any part of the body.

On the other hand, gonorrhoea is known to be

caused by a specific micro-organism 'Gonococcus', which affects, especially the urethra and vagina. The incubation period ranges from two to ten days. In the absence of treatment the infection almost always extends deeper to involve the posterior part of urethra, the neck of the bladder and the prostate gland. Arthritis is the most common of the extra genital manifestations of gonorrhoea. Gonococcal endocarditis (involvement of the heart valves) is, however, responsible for almost all of the fatalities caused by gonorrhoea.

It is, however, worthwhile to mention here that at least three more distinct varieties of venereal diseases are there, namely — 'Lymphogranuloma venereum', 'Granuloma inguinale' and 'Chancroid', caused by distinctly different causative organisms. Of these granuloma inguinale is known to be extremely chronic. The course of lymphogranuloma venereum, caused by a virus, is also known to vary from a symptomatic infection to extreme debility with chronic invalidism as a result of late manifestation[41].

Hahnemann observed that we must confess that the expulsion of a few vesicles of itch, that have just arisen, often shows no immediate, manifestly strong, evil consequences, but the more months a neglected itch eruption has flourished on the skin, the more surely the internal psora which underlies it has been able to reach a great degree, with dangerous consequences[9].

One recent finding in molecular biology is that, while mutations may arise in any type of cell carrying inheritable material, if one occurs in cells which give rise only to somatic tissue, the mutation will be eliminated with the death of the individual. If however, the mutation occurs in a cell which gives rise to germ tissue, it can pass from one generation to the next. This conforms with the homoeopathic observation that the susceptibility of psora, sycosis and syphilis is laid by inheritance and that the complicated forms of psora are those which are inherited.

For descriptive purposes, mutant genes have been grouped into three distinct categories, viz., 'lethal', 'semi-lethal' and 'sub-lethal', based on the effect they have on the phenotype. This may remind one of the three categories of chronic miasm, — syphilis', 'sycosis' and 'psora', which are different in producing their distinctly different effects on the body.

While psora is more commonly known to attack the blood vessels and liver, and causes deposits beneath the skin, forming suppuration and boils, sycosis affects the soft tissues, and syphilis affects both the soft tissues and the bones[42].

In recent time J.N. Kanjilal put forward a more comprehensive description of the same. He observed that, 'psora' is the sensitizing miasm, producing no structural change but only functional disorder, manifested by hypersensitivity, —itching, irritation, burning, utmost up to congestion and inflammation. 'Sycosis' is (the incoordination miasm producing inco-ordination everywhere, mental or physical, and syphilis is the destructive miasm producing destructive disorder everywhere, mental or physical.

Whatsoever it may be, the three chronic miasms seem to indicate or symbolize the three distinctly different categories of gene mutation, creating thereby certain conditions in the system that give rise to specific types of diseases, each in its own way. Psora symbolizing sub-lethal (sensitizing), sycosis semi-lethal (inco-ordinating) and syphilis lethal (destructive) type of mutation.

Normal development is known to be highly sensitive process and depends on the harmoniously integrated function of thousands of genic units, changes or loss of which through mutation may lead to a breakdown of development. Expression of emotional disorder is also said to be closely linked with a genetic background.

It has also been observed, gene generally produces more of visible effects on the individual, while there may be many invisible effects also of the same gene, and in case where a condition of susceptibility to certain disease is present, it may be that a careful scrutiny will detect some minor visible effects produced by the same gene.

While spontaneous mutations are found to occur under natural conditions of environment, mutation may also be produced by various physical and chemical agents and are known as induced mutations. While no chemical agents of sufficiently low toxicity are available for treatment of systematic bacterial infection, various drugs including penicillin are known to give rise to extensive and persistent urticaria. In fact there are literally thousands of natural and synthetic chemicals which are capable of sensitizing the human skin.

Superficial bacterial infection is also known to give rise to chronic kidney disturbances, due lo absorption of toxic agents produced by the organism.

It may, therefore, be observed that diseases involving gene mutation, spontaneous or induced under influence of some prolonged stimuli are 'chronic' in nature, while on the other hand 'acute' diseases do not involve any structural defect or gene mutation and are caused only by temporary functional defects in the defense mechanism of the body.

It is interesting to note in this context that certain substances such as coffee, tobacco etc. are known to create hindrances to quick recovery' in chronic diseases. This is possibly because coffee contains 'caffeine' and tobacco contains 'carcinogen', both the substances being intensely mutagenic, may have adverse influences on the concerned genes, creating thereby hindrances to recovery. Similarly many chemicals and drug substances having mutagenic property may have to be stopped or restricted during homoeopathic treatment, particularly of chronic diseases.

10. Systematics of Prescribing

The four fundamentals of homoeopathy as laid down by Hahnemann in his 'Organon of Medicine are the proving of substances to be used as medicines, the selection and administration of the so proved medicine according to the law of similimum, the single remedy and the minimum dose.

At a rough guess, some two or three thousand remedies are in use in homoeopathy and new ones are being continually developed. But only a small fraction of these has been thoroughly proved in accordance with the Hahnemannian standard. More-over, toxicological data and also the results obtained from clinical experiments have been included into the 'Materia Medica', which made it liable to criticism[43], because sickness not only modifies the responses of organism to drugs, but also no true 'drug picture' can be obtained from the sick.

Experiments with crude drugs are also not preferred as they fail to produce finer reactions. Then again, though the main criteria emphasized in homoeopathy is the use of remedies exactly on experimentations, that is, provings on healthy human beings and also individualization of the patient to which the individualization of the remedy responds, yet many so-called homoeopathic remedies are known to be empirically used and some are claimed to be disease specifics.

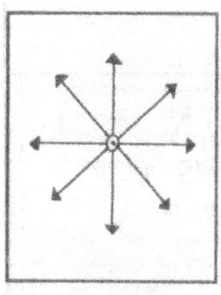

Figure 10.1

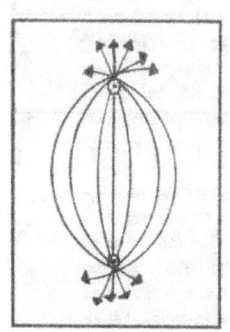

Figure 10.2

Philosophically the word 'holism' means wholes, that are more than the sum of the parts, while 'individualism' means an individual peculiarity. The two words, although apparently contradictory, have tremendous significance in selection of homoeopathic remedies.

Although Hahnemann specifically stressed on the totality of symptoms, clearly mentioning in aphorism-18 of the Organon of Medicine, 'that the sum of all the symptoms and conditions in each individual case of disease must be the sole indication, the sole guide to direct us in the choice of a remedy, yet the importance of the phrase has not been properly understood by many.

The underlying meaning of the phrase 'totality of symptoms' is most uniquely expressed through the single word 'holism'. It clarifies beyond all doubts that the totality of symptoms can neither be mere conglomeration nor the numerical sum of all the symptoms. But it is in reality something more than the sum total, the symptomatic wholeness of the patient's image. A simple example may clarify the point.

Suppose there is a 'flower vase' on the table with various beautiful flowers arranged in it. If you are shown only a small part of it, keeping the remaining portions under cover, it becomes absolutely difficult for you to guess the whole object.

But as soon as the cover is removed, the flower vase appears before you in totality and you get a clear picture of the same. But still then you are seeing only the half portion of the object and that too from a particular angle. Yet that makes no difference and you are able to portray the other half and visualize the object in its entirety, that is in wholeness. This is what is meant by 'holism'.

Then again 'holism', although apparently seems to be contradictory to 'individualism', both are in reality complementary to each other. Thus the uncommon individualistic symptoms instead of getting rejected by the totality of symptoms in fact become the very basis of the latter. While totality of symptoms is the sole guide to find out a whole image, the specificity of the image lies in uncommon peculiar and characteristic symptoms.

A graphical representation of the symptom syndrome may be the best possible way to find out a similimum.

Suppose we are given a single point. We can draw innumerable lines out of the point to all possible directions (Figure 10.1), Similarly with a single symptom, notwithstanding its singularity or peculiarity, we often remain confused having a number of remedies against it. Thus 'aggravation in the morning', may indicate as many as seventy-five remedies starting from 'Aconite' to '

Veratrum'. Given with two points the direction is to some extent restricted, but still then we are confused whether the line should be a curve or a straight line (Figure 10,2).

It is only when we are given with a minimum of three points, we are in a definite position to draw a specific line or graph (Figure 10.3).

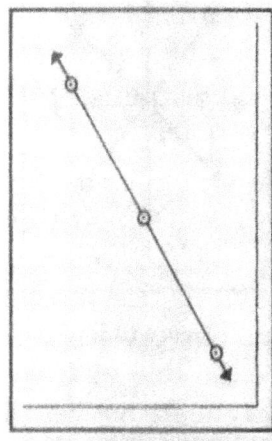

Figure 10.3

The well known 'three legged stool' (location, sensation and modalities) theory of Hering should possibly be viewed from this angle.

Then again we should not forget that a graph is only a specific indication of a particular trend and it is not necessary that it should pass through all the points collected. It should only touch the salient points so that the trend is properly indicated and may leave aside the rest on either sides of the line at various distances (Figure 10.4).

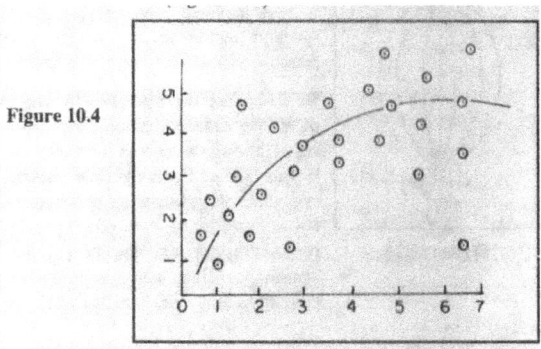

Figure 10.4

Thus to select a specific homoeopathic remedy out of a given symptom syndrome, it is not necessary that each and every symptom is to be taken into account, but only those which may he found to specifically represent the general trend of the symptom syndrome.

Although there seems to exist two distinctly different schools, represented by the so-called 'unicists' and 'pluralists Hahnemann himself insisted on giving just one remedy at a time, because the materia medica provings were thus carried out.

Use of multiple remedies at a time may not only alter or hinder one another's action but also create additional drug stimulus, confusing thereby the whole issue. Hence it was observed that use of multiple remedies at a time cannot cure the ailment profoundly and permanently, even if each of the remedies might be capable of wiping out the fragmentary illness for which they were applied, further, it was observed that the effect of the multiple remedies may not be necessarily the sum total of the effects of the individual remedies, but rather a combination function as a single remedy and therefore would require separate proving.

In employing homoeopathic remedies in potencies, the size of dose is said to be immaterial. But there is some division in practice as to whether the remedy should be used in single or multiple doses and their repeatability. As a general practice, the lower potencies are used in repeated doses in acute cases, while the higher potencies are used in single dose in chronic cases over a longer period.

Hahnemann himself is said to have approved repetition of doses at definite intervals, provided the degree of each dose deviates somewhat from the preceding and following ones. Consequently Dishingten discovered 'plus dosage' where successive doses are slightly elevated. M. Tyler and Renand introduced 'fractional dosage' whereby a dose is broken into three parts and administered at one hourly intervals. Gordon promulgated 'double dosage' in which two doses of the same remedy but at different potencies are administered at eight hourly intervals i.e. at bedtime and on rising, the lower potency being followed by the higher potency a general rule, however, the frequency of the doses is said to be dependent on the amelioration or aggravation of the situation[44], although there are practitioners who are known to prescribe the same remedy frequently and continually for a prolonged period[45].

Selection of potencies is said to be the most difficult and puzzling problem in homoeopathy. Although different homoeopaths based on their practicing experience promulgated different rules and guidelines, unfortunately these all led to more confusion and none could be universally acceptable [46].

Hahnemann during his lifetime used generally up to 30 centesimal' potency and rarely used higher, although at the fag end of his life he introduced the LM (50-millesimal) potencies. The basic difference of the fifty-millesimal potency with that of centesimal potency is that, in case of fifty-millesimal potency, at every stage the strength of diluent is increased from hundred to fifty thousand and the number of succussion is increased from ten to hundred. So, on the one hand the crude drug molecules are eliminated more quickly in the process of dilution and on the other hand the rate of formation of light isotopic molecules is enhanced in the process of increased number of succussion.

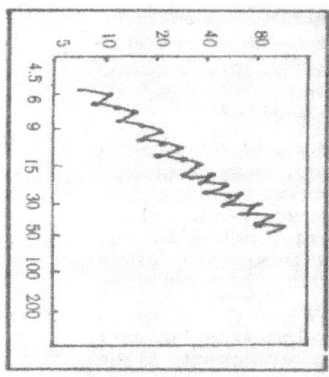

Figure 10.5

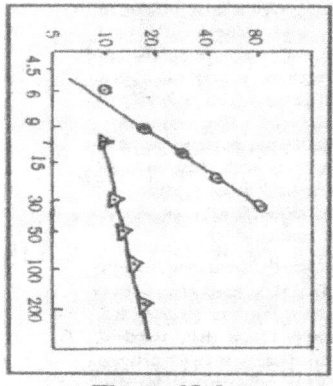

Figure 10.6

Moreover, though in both the cases the strength of potency advances following a sine cure (wave like motion), yet in case of Fifty-millesimal potency it will be more intensified and sharp in character (Figure 10.5). So if separate graphs are drawn then the lines connecting the peak points will be found distinctly different in nature. In case of centesimal potency the line will be almost parallel to the abscissa only being slightly inclined, whereas in case of fifty millesimal potency it will be found sharply inclined toward the ordinate, showing sharp rise in the strength of potency (Figure 10.6). So we see in case of fifty millesimal potency there is marked differences in strength at short frequencies, whereas one has to use potencies in leaps and bounds in case of centesimal potency.

Thus it is apparent that in fifty - millesimal potency, medicines may be administered almost continuously and in quick succession, particularly in acute diseases, without the risk of marked aggravation of the disease symptoms and at the same time greatly shortening the total lime of recovering period.

Since the beginning, however, the homoeopathic world was found to be divided into two groups, the low potentists' and the 'high potentists'[47].

Hughes. Boyd, Price, Ritter and others were know as supporters of low potencies because high potencies were supposed to contain no drug molecule, while Kent, Boenninghausen, Nash and the followers were advocates of high potencies and believed that the low potency group was solely responsible for the downfall of homoeopathy in many of the advanced western countries[47].

Case, Barker, Gordon and others were however or the opinion that there is a *homoeopathicity* in the potency as in the remedy and until the potency is adjusted to the plane of the individual during illness (i.e. optimum potency) the remedy does not become similimum. But Allen, Brown and Ward believed that any potency would work if the remedy is selected on similimum. Suggestions were also put forward for the selection of homoeopathic potencies in accordance with the nature of the disease, sensitivity of the patient, constitution, temperament etc. Some homoeopaths even observed that where pathological symptoms predominate lower potencies are indicated and for diseases of manifestly psychic origin higher potencies may be needed[46].

It is however generally believed that the lower potencies act quickly and superficially and therefore should be used in acute cases, while higher potencies act slowly and deeply and as such they are needed in chronic cases[45]. But there are others who believe that the potencies do not have any relevance to the depth and speed of action[48].

Following observation of J.T. Kent seems to be of primary importance in systematizing homoeopathic prescribing, — "We have thus two things to deal with the 'acute' and the 'chronic' states. The acute miasm being very opposite in character and order to the chronic miasm. The fact that the homoeopathic physicians must know is, that which is true in many respects in acute case may be the very opposite in a chronic case[42]."

In this context it is interesting to note that the genetic effect of radiation is related to dose, the frequency of mutation being directly and simply proportional to the dose. At one time it was believed that the effect was the same whether the dose was given in a short time or separated out over a long period. But recent experiments on mice have shown that the effect of a single exposure is greater than the effect of the same dose administered as several smaller doses separated by the interval of time [16]. So it may be inferred that in acute cases comparatively lower potencies of the short acting remedy may be repeated frequently until the favourable reaction starts, because in such cases the specific (antigen- antibody like) immunological response is to be stimulated. Whereas in case of chronic disease, a single dose of the high potency deep-acting remedy is to be administered and a long wait for the reverse mutation response to start.

Further, the mutation frequency was found to differ with different genetic stocks and also in different portions of the natural life-cycle of the same individual. This corroborates with the homoeopathic observation that, different potencies act differently not only in different cases but also with the same individual at different times and conditions.

Hahnemann, Kent and others insisted that the doses must be consistent with the degree of susceptibility or sensitivity of the patient. In other words, the higher the sensitivity of the patient the milder should be the homoeopathic dose and the vice-versa. Thus in case of children, who are generally very sensitive and also in cases of oversensitive patients, milder doses (6c to 200c potencies) may be given, while in cases of sluggish and poorly sensitive patients stronger doses (above 200c potencies) may be used.

The frequency of the doses is said to be dependent on the nature of the disease as well as the gravity of the situation. The author is of the opinion that the repeatability of the doses is inversely proportional to the sensitivity of the patient. Hence in highly sensitive patients notwithstanding milder doses repetition may not be required, while in poorly sensitive patients in spite of stronger doses frequent repetition may be necessary for initiating reaction.

However, it is to be specifically noted in this connection that the repetition of doses beyond their homoeopathicity, especially in cases of over-sensitive or feeble patients, may sometimes establish a miasm, imitating a chronic or acute one, in accordance with the ability of the drug[42].

Although genetically controlled immunological system is known to be highly specific, there exist some 'near specifics' depending on the closeness of relation. Hence in homoeopathic prescribing the remedies on 'near similimum' may also be administered, the effectiveness of which will depend on the greatest similarity to the totality of symptoms. Thus it is not indispensable that all the symptoms of the drug correspond to all the symptoms of the patient, neither it is possible, given the infinite richness of human symptomatology and of the experimental symptomatology.

It has also been observed that not only a chronic patient may be suffering from an acute miasm but also all the three chronic miasms psora, sycosis and syphilis may be mixed up together, it is therefore important to avoid getting confused by two or more disease images that may exist in the body at the same time. Because any attempt to cure them all by collecting the symptoms that the patient has had in a life-time and thereby prescribing on totality of symptoms is bound to result in error.

It is important to note in this context that as per some recent finding the immunological defects may arise simultaneously with gene-mutation and also different types of mutations i.e. lethal, semi-lethal and sub-lethal may concurrently occur in the system. Also it has been observed that not only different mutations occurring at the same locus can lead to important results but also the way in which genes change as a result of successive mutations remains to be gone into in greater length[49].

Then again different miasms when mixed up together, only one of them is found to be predominant and disease producing at a given time, while the others remain dormant and inactive. The nature and influence of a particular miasm is also found to be dependent on its first acquisition, and the one arising from heredity is said to be most characteristic by its depth and slowness.

On consideration of above facts and observations it is therefore essential that the physician should choose only those symptoms which are most expressive and predominant, evaluate them with equal importance and finally individualize things widely dissimilar in one way although similar in other ways. We should also collect the background history of the patient so that a direction of how to proceed stepwise is obtained.

It has been observed that the recent symptoms are indicative of active disturbance and are of the highest prescribing value, while the remote symptoms are those which might have occurred in the past and are only called to mind on thorough enquiry. They point to remedies that might have been prescribed at the time and are of value even now if administered[44].

Kent observed that the worst symptoms should be singled out and covered carefully with a remedy ignoring entirely the other ones. Then as these disappear the ones that have remained, become more and more apparent from day to day, when ultimately a second remedy may be required.

Hahnemann also advised that after each new dose of remedy has exhausted its action and is no longer suitable and helpful, the state of the disease that still remains is to be noted anew with respect to its remaining symptoms and another homoeopathic remedy sought for, as suitable as possible, for the group of symptoms now observed, and so on until the recovery is complete. Thus in chronic case either involving mutations to single gene or multiple genes, it is always probable that symptoms will reappear in the reverse order of their coming.

Mutations occurring due to addition or subtraction of one or more bases from the genetic message cannot however be reversed by 'mutagenes', because these can only change one base into another. Hahnemann also recognized the possibility of presence of advanced irreversible pathological tissue damage which cannot be reversed by homoeopathic remedies[44].

11. Homoeopathy in Cancer Treatment

Cancer is an autonomous new growth of tissues of an unknown basic cause. In case of cancer, one or more cells suddenly begin to grow by division at a rate which may approximate or equal to that which normally occur before birth.

Such centres of growth known as tumours, may show different degrees of disorganization and lack of control. Some, such as warts, wens and moles, ordinarily cease growth without intervention or treatment and are called 'benign'. Others classified as 'malignant' continue with unabated vigour and invade surrounding tissues by direct or contagious growth or it may infiltrate within blood and lymph vessels in which the cells are broken off and carried to distant organs in which they lodge through filtrate, a process known as metastasis.

Although as yet there is no unambiguous evidence that any class of human cancer is regularly caused by a virus, the possibility that C type RNA tumour viruses are involved in human neoplastic disease has been the subject of much speculation and experimentation in recent times In particular human leukaemia has come under close scrutiny because many cases of leukaemia in diverse species of anima's have a viral aetiology[51].

One of the most reasonable theory of the origin of

cancer postulates that several genes in each cell independently restrain it from forming a cancer, so that until each of those genes has been inactivated by mutation, it will not form one.

Mutations can be induced either by environ-mental mutagens or arise as a spontaneous error during replication of DNA at any time in the life of a cell. Most forms of human cancer seem from their age indication to be the end result of several mutational steps that may have taken place at any time in the patient's life.

The total incubation period of any cancer therefore is countable from the moment when the first step took place, presumably some 10 to 20 years back. There are however hundred or so distinct varieties of cancer (Figure 11.1).

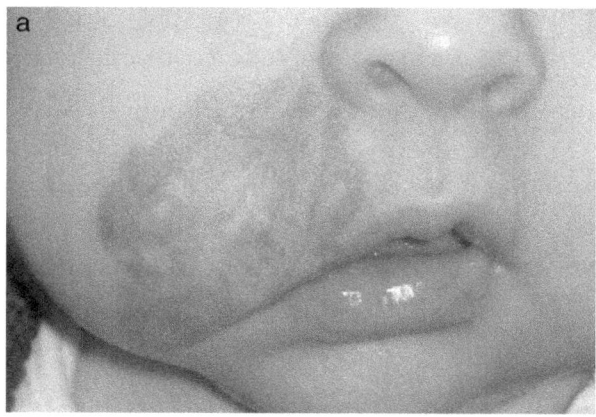

Figure 11.1 (A case of haemangioma of face)

The dichotomy between 'viral' and 'genetic' theories

of the origin of cancer has however been resolved recently with the discovery concerning the interaction between 'tumour virus' and the 'genetic material' of the cell. It is now believed that the elements related to viral RNA are attached to the 'genome' of the cell and transmitted genetically to become activated at some future time and cause spontaneous cancer[52].

Though the mechanism by which cancer cells form is not yet fully known, the number of newly discovered 'carcinogens' (agents which induce formation of cancer) continues to increase every day. The three general classes of carcinogens recognized are radiations, chemicals and viruses.

The history of cancer by chemical carcinogens dates back to 1915, when long-term application of coal tar on the ears of rabbits was found to produce cancer. In 1930 cancer was also produced on the skin of mice by application of a pure polycyclic aromatic hydrocarbon.

Thus while cancer malady is believed to be the end result of several consecutive mutations, certain chronic stimuli, such as X-ray, radium, some chemicals (present in pitch, tar etc.) are known to produce degenerative changes in the skin which may result in cancer.

There are more than four hundred chemical substances called 'carcinogen', which when introduced on the animal by painting the skin or into the animal by subcutaneous or intraperitoneal injection, are often followed by a reaction on the part of the animal which results in cancer formation.

The technique for the production of skin cancer

consisted in applying the substance in benzene solution (0.3 g in 100 ml) to the interscapular region of mice twice weekly. Tests for the production of 'sarcoma' were made by injecting the compound in fatty medium such as lard.

Results of animal experiments show that '3:4 – benzphenanthrene' is the simplest hydrocarbon having carcinogenic activity, and the most powerful carcinogenic agent so far discovered is methylchlolathrene'. Other types of chemical carcinogens identified include various 'azocompounds', 'aromatic amines', 'aminostilbenes', 'nitrogen mustards', 'urethanes', various 'aliphatic compounds', 'epoxides' and a few inorganic salts.

By mid-20th century many inorganic and organic compounds had been recognized as capable of causing cancer in humans by occupational hazard (Figure 11.2).

The quantity of these agents may be so minute as not to cause apparent irritation during the time of exposure.

The change is gradually induced in the tissue which ultimately becomes cancerous. The precancerous change may be so permanent that malignant tumour may develop many years after the particular occupation has been abandoned.

It is interesting to note in this context that the most powerful experimental carcinogens are also known to be intensely mutagenic[53].

For the vast majority of cancers there is no specific drug as yet and the results obtained so far from treatments by surgery, radiation and cytotoxic drugs are not very encouraging. Fewer than half of all cancer

Occupational Carcinogens	Type of cancer produced
Benzol	Leukaemia
Aniline, benzidine,	Pipilomas
Chrome salts, nickel-carbonyl and asbestos dust	Cancer of the respiratory tract
Pitch, Coal tar, Crude paraffins, Crude minerral oils and arsenic compounds	Multiple cancers involving the skin, Chiefly of the hands, arms and scrotum.
2- naphthylamine	Bladder cancer
Benzpyrene	Lung cancer
Radio active metal paints	Bone sarcoma

Figure 11.2

Appearance of cancer in old age shows that simply the immune system is failing. The association of malignancy with impaired immunity also suggests that improving the immune response may be beneficial in some type of cancer. Moreover, it is again in virus diseases that the production of immunity by vaccination has been most successful, since virus attack specific tissues in the body and multiply within cells, they cannot be reacted on by antibiotics, which are administered via blood serum.

Surgery and radiation, most widely used in cancer treatment, are said to be maximally effective only when the cancer is localized. If the cancer cells are disseminated throughout the body, therapy is required that would reach and destroy them. This being the chief advantage of chemotherapy, all cancer chemotherapeutic agents are, however, known to be injurious to normal cells, which fact places limits on their ultimate effectiveness.

The fourth kind of cancer treatment is popularly known as immunotherapy. The principal attractiveness of immunotherapy lies in the extraordinary specificity of immunological reactions. It is, therefore, thought that the destruction of cancer cells marked by specific antigens may accomplished without injuring the normal cells lacking those antigens.

Vast amount of work is being carried out in different laboratories and clinics around the world, to apply immunological principles to the treatment of malignancy, although at the moment there is said to be no comparable regime of immunotherapy with predictable benefit to the cancer patient, excepting only some hints of what the future will hold.

Alkylating agents like 'nitrogen mustard', 'cyclophosphamide', etc. known as anti-cancer drugs have proved to be effective inhibitor of tumour growth, but these so-called 'radio mimetic' agents have frequently been shown to be carcinogenic. Paradoxically again, though radiation is used to treat cancer, it is also known to induce cancer.

This indicates that doses and methods of application are the main factors in determining the effect of the agents used, which in turn indicates that the carcinogens possibly contain the nucleus of cures for cancer, by following the famous homoeopathic dictum, 'similia similibus curentur'.

Certain benign tumours, which are known to be precancerous in varying percentages and may degenerate into malignant forms, are already known to be responsive to homoeopathic system of treatment (Figure 11.3). Moreover, warts are particularly common complication in patients with primary and secondary immunodeficiencies and in patients under immunosuppression, which respond definitely and curatively to homoeopathic potentized medicines.

So homoeopathy is possibly the required form of immunotherapy, which may be most effectively directed against the disorganized and invasive behaviour of cancer cells. A big field is awaiting homoeopathic exploration and even the slightest success would be a great boon to the suffering humanity.

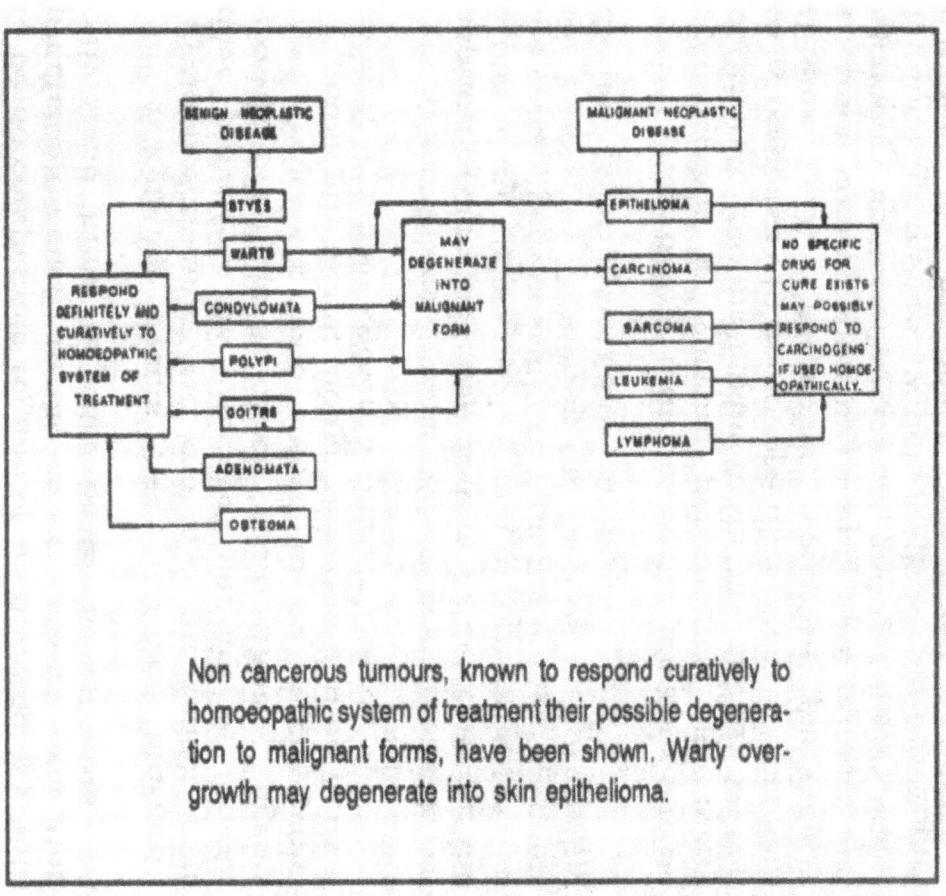

Figure 11.3

It would be a simple step to potentize the particular carcinogens and conduct some clinical experiments. The crucial knowledge as regards to carcinogens producing particular cancer is already available through animal experimentations as well as occupational hazards. One has only got to compile them systematically and direct the same towards a meaningful purpose.

12. Homoeopathy in Population Control

In the year 1798, T.R.Malthus, an English clergyman and economist was first to express his concern with the world's expanding population which would outrun the food supply, leading mankind to outbreed itself into starvation and poverty. In spite of the checks due to the widespread of Europe nearly doubled, in the span of a mere hundred years, between the 1750's and 1850's.

In the pre-Malthusian period however the three terrible trio – warm, famine and epidemic ensured a steady and substantial check on population growth. With the advancements in hygiene and sanitation in most developed and developing countries, man has, however, reversed all these natural control and the life expectancy has nearly doubled, without having concurrent check on the birth rate. Thus while mortality is falling, fertility has remained at a high level and the exceedingly rapid rate of population growth has made the socio-economic conditions in many countries quit explosive (Figure 12.1).

WORLD POPULATION INCRASE	
Year	Population
1850	1 billion
1925	2 billion
1964	3 billion
1980	4 billion
1990	5 billion
2000	6 billion
2020	7.8 billion

Figure 12.1

In all societies, some sort of attempts, conscious or unconscious, were known to control human fertility. Ritual restrictions on the frequency of relation between sexes, postponement of marriage, induced abortion, infanticide or the exposure of unwanted infants were found to be practiced. Lactation period was also known to be prolong in some primitive societies with the belief that it would reduce the chances of conception. Artificial interference with conception is however, known to be widely practiced only in modern societies.

Francis Place, a London tailor and labour leader, in 1822, for the first time, decried the burden of large families upon people of limited means and advocated the use of contraception techniques. The move was however, resisted as usual on moral and ethical grounds by the state machineries and the religious institutions.

In 1833, Charles Knowlton of Boston was fined and jailed for bringing in public the knowledge of the medical profession on contraception. In 1877, a generation later, in England, Annie Besant was tried on a charge of immorality for republication of the Knowlton tract. In 1916, the first U.S. birth control clinic opened by Margaret in Brooklyn was raided and closed by police, Mrs. Sanger receiving a 30 days' imprisonment.

By mid-20th century, legal restrictions against contraception where virtually disappearing, although by 1975, Connecticut and Massachusetts continued to enforce laws forbidding a physician to offer contraceptive information to a married woman patient for whom pregnancy might be injurious or even fatal. Today, however, the situation is quite different and governments of many countries recognize the present rate of population growth (Figure 12.2) as a stumbling block to a rise in their people's standard of living.

> DEATHS BY NATURAL CALAMITIES
>
> Natural calamities such as earth quakes, floods, cyclones and tornadoes kill thousands of people every year in several parts of the world.
>
> In a recent cyclone in Bangladesh over 50,000 people were killed. But with a birth-rate of 3.3 per cent per years, the number was replaced in just 40 days!

Figure 12.2

Birth control is achieved at present either by introducing some barrier, mechanical or chemical, to prevent effective meeting of the male sperm (Figure 12.3) and the ovum (Figure 12.4 & 12.5) , or through self-imposed restraints such as withdrawal or limiting coition to the safe period.

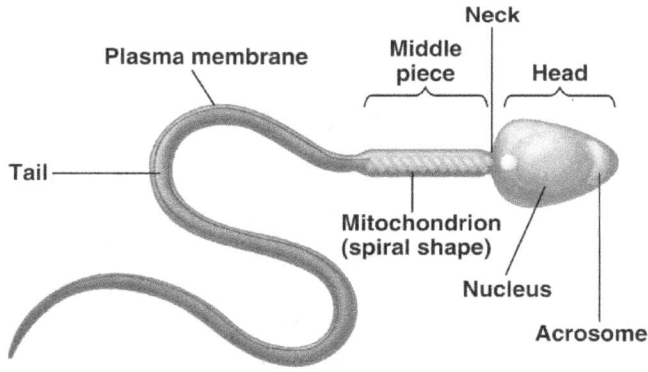

Figure 12.3

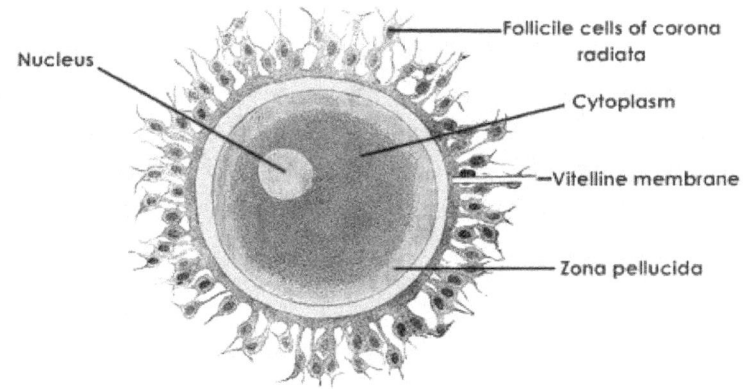

Figure 12.4

Although research into family planning has expanded considerably in the past fifteen years and many methods of contraception are available, yet hardly any of them is universally acceptable, on cultural, political and medical consideration[54]. The low initial acceptor rates and high discontinuation for present methods is undoubtedly indicative of a pressing need for new methods to be developed[55].

The 'safe period' method is complicated is risky, and the methods of 'withdrawal' is difficult and may cause great harm if practiced carelessly for a long period. The 'intra-uterine-devices' (IUD) require a scarce measure of skill and the 'condoms' are not so reliable. In spite of effectiveness the 'pills' may have serious side effects and are also inconvenient due to their once-a-day regimen. Post coital pills or Morning after Pills (To be taken within 72 hours of unprotected sex) are extremely unsafe and not recommended for regular use as well.

'Surgical sterilization' on the other hand is more drastic and at the same time irrevocable, 'Abortion' in early pregnancy, although effective to a good extent due to development of various techniques e.g. vacuum suction, menstrual regulation (MR) etc., is not a contraceptive measure in true sense. Moreover, it requires continuous medical or paramedical supervision, since serious complications like post-abortion bleeding, blood coagulation disorder etc. are known to arise. Further, it is to be noted that scientists are yet to invent an oral abortifacient[56].

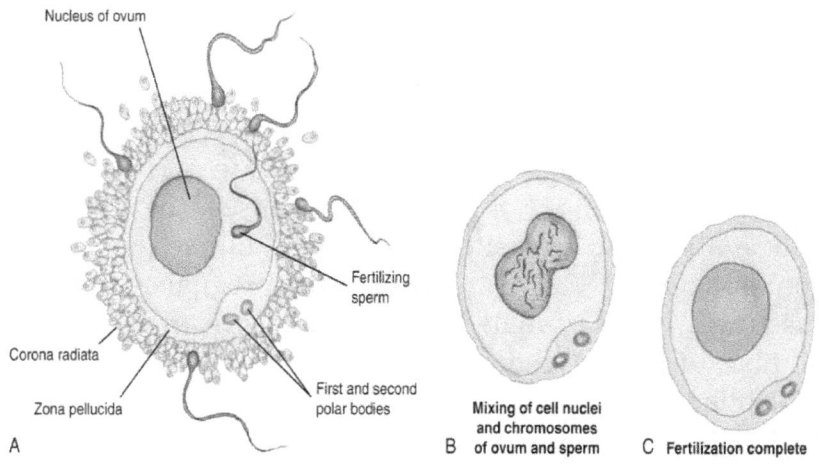

Figure 12.5(a)

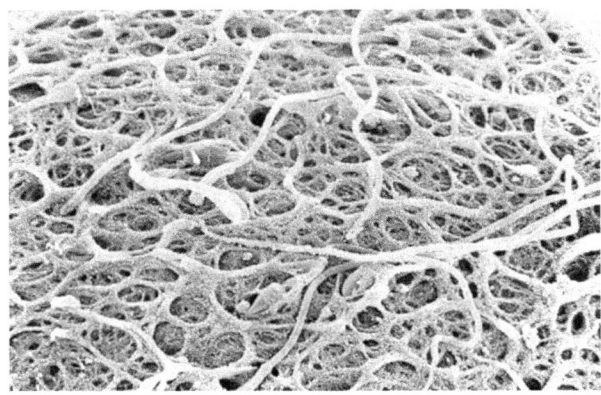

Figure 12.5(b)

The fact that human hormones can be made 'antigenic' in the human, opened up the possibilities of immunological control of fertility[54].

It has been known that 'Follicle stimulating hormone' (FSH) causes an egg-containing follicle in the ovary to ripen; 'Luteinising hormone (LH) causes the ripened follicle to burst releasing the egg'; 'Human chorionic gonadotrophin' (HCG) causes the pregnancy to be sustained. Thus female reproductive system offers a number of points where the reproductive process can be controlled e.g. ovulation, transport of the egg, transport of the sperm, fertilization and implantation[57].

Clinical trials of anti-pregnancy vaccine are already under way in India and abroad. The vaccine is supposed to trigger an immune response by producing anti-bodies to either 'HCG" or the 'Zona Pellucida' of the matured egg and thereby preventing conception[58]. It is, however, feared that the use of such vaccines may affect other physiological functions, including the subsequent pregnancy and the health of future offspring, due to probable cross reactivity. Reversibility of such vaccines are also under serious doubt.

Homoeopathic system of treatment being closely related with the immune response mechanism of the body, naturally the question may arise whether homoeopathy has anything to contribute to the concept of immunological control of fertility.

So far in homoeopathy, medicines like Natrum mur, Lycopodium, Pulsatilla etc. are said to be prescribed for contraceptive purposes. These well proved medicines are known to produce some kind of sterility, impotence or even abortion, when administered in toxic doses. It is to be noted in this context that homoeopathic medicines used in toxic- doses may cause even greater damage, as they are supposed to work on deeper dynamic level.

Therefore, if the theory of 'Similia similibus curentur' is to be applied for inhibition of fertility, then systematic homoeopathic researches are to be carried out to mimic the physiological state found during the periods of natural infertility in women, with synthetic or natural human hormones responsible for fertility and conception.

The birth control measures are abnormal and unnatural processes and the womenfolk may be ill-adapted to spend the greater part of their reproductive lives in the non-pregnant state, brought about either by internal medicinal contraceptives or by any other means. But since there is no way out and birth control measures being a pressing need of the present socio-economic condition, it may be wise to adopt a harmless form, rather than to expose mankind to harmful and mechanical measures.

If the physiological state found in women during the periods of natural infertility i.e. pregnancy, lactation or before puberty could be re-established homoeopathically in a controllable manner without any harmful side effect, it would be the most universally acceptable method for family planning.

Meanwhile, the fact that the homoeopathic system of medicament fulfils all the preconditions necessary for an ideal contraceptive[59], being cheap, convenient, long-lasting, reversible, harmless and at the same time free from continuous medical supervision cannot be denied.

13.
Homoeopathy in Plant Pathology

Diseases of plants are known from time immemorial. It is, however, in recent times that their study, particularly of cultivated plants, has been taken up in an organized and scientific manner. Now-a-days it is known that most of the plant diseases result from the invasion of the plant tissues by bacteria, fungi, viruses etc. In the absence of any parasite, the disease symptoms may also be produced due to certain physical or chemical features of the environment.

Plant diseases, particularly caused by different pathogens, are mainly responsible for present in-creasing imbalance between the world's need for food and the amount available. Diseases caused by fungi alone annually destroy food that could have fed three hundred million people. The damage caused by plant diseases becomes most striking and devastating when it comes on in an epidemic form. The 'wheat rust' of Prussia in 1891, the 'potato blight' of Ireland in 1846, and the 'coffee leaf disease' of Ceylon in 1870 are some of the glaring examples.

To control plant diseases methods generally adopted are directed either to destroy the parasites by insecticides, fungicides, crop rotation etc. or to develop resistant varieties of plants. Most of the control measures have, however, their limitations and disadvantages.

Crop rotation is effective only against short lived invaders and fallowing or eradication is uneconomical. Insecticides and fungicides are absorbed by the plant and accumulated in the fat of animals and human beings. Also 'pests' gradually evolve a strain more resistant to the material, so that the strength has to be increased or a new material found. Developing resistant varieties is slow and continuous process. Moreover, a new variety can itself be a hazard or cease to work at any moment.

Further, it has been observed that plants may show deficiency disease due to lack of some important chemical constituents. The lack of magnesium, potassium, iron, copper, zinc etc. are known to produce characteristic chlorosis, in which 'chlorophyll', the green pigment of the plant, fails to develop properly. The disease symptoms are, however, known to be corrected or cured by addition of the substances in the soil, in 'macro' or 'micronutrient' forms.

Conversely, disease conditions are also said to result from the presence of an excess of certain chemicals in the soil. Thus various kinds of chlorosis may also be caused due to excess of calcium, magnesium, potassium etc.

It is also known that substances may exert important and beneficial physiological effects when present in infinitesimally small and undetectable amount, but when the amounts are increased, although in a very small proportion, they become harmful to plants[60]. Not only inorganic matters but also organic substances like auxins

Homoeopathy in the Light of Modern Science

in low concentrations are known to produce toxic effects, while in very dilute solution they provoke characteristic growth response in plants[61].

It is further known that in spite of being a poisonous element very low concentration of 'arsenic' is beneficial to plants, producing noticeable stimulation of growth which is believed to result from some sort of catalytic action[62], and certain plants respond to 'sodium', although a non-essential element.

Although the essential elements are known to correct the specific disease symptoms in plants, known as deficiency symptoms, the exact role of many of these elements are still unknown"[61]. Moreover, the similar disease symptoms are known to be produced by a great variety of causes. Wilting of foliage, for example, may occur due to damage of the root by fungal or insect attack. Various degree of discolorization of leaves resembling zinc or iron deficiency are also known to be caused by micoplasma, a plant disease agent[63].

With the discovery of micro-nutrients (trace elements), a large number of hitherto obscure plant diseases were identified as micro-nutrient deficiencies[64]. But it became difficult to reconcile how the similar disease symptoms could be developed by substances in toxic level. It is to be noted in this context that a common character of all the micro-nutrients is that they are needed in very small quantity and they become toxic if present in larger quantities in available form[65].

The lack of some 'macro-nutrients' (major elements) such as calcium, magnesium, potassium etc. is also known to produce characteristic chlorosis, while the same disease conditions are known to result from their presence in toxic level[66].

It is however known that the plants are less responsive with increasing age and the germination stage is particularly known to be highly sensitive to adverse environmental conditions[65].

To examine the phenomena some experiments were conducted by the authors on wheat plants, in distilled water culture, with some essential elements (macro, as well as, micro-nutrients) in homoeopathic potencies. The purpose of the experiments was to see whether toxicity symptoms could be produced by the substances in homoeopathic dilutions (particularly beyond the Avogadro's limit) and also to study the exact nature of the symptoms produced.

Details of the experiments were as follows: Different glass pots of uniform size and shape were taken. To each pot one ounce of distilled water was poured. Different substances in homoeopathic potencies were added to the water in drop doses and stirred well. To these a few numbers of wheat seeds collected from the same stock was allowed to soak overnight. The excess water was then decanted out and the seeds were allowed to germinate. After germination the seeds were picked up and three replications of each were made and then allowed the plants to grow in distilled water culture. The atmospheric temperature during the experiment was about 80° F.

Since fourth day after germination the plants grown

in water culture, particularly treated with high homoeopathic potencies (1M or 1000c) started showing symptoms of disease or toxicity. By the tenth day symptoms were almost fully developed.

On critical examination it was found that the disease symptoms produced by the homoeopathic potencies (Figure 13.) of substances were identical to their deficiency symptoms (Figure 13.2) known60. Whereas, by post-germination treatment growth simulation effects were only observed (Figure13.3). It was of particular interest to note that with Cuprum sulphuricum, both 6c and 1M potencies, the growth of leaves were stunted with tips having lost colour and inclined to die. Whereas with Ferrum sulphuricum, in same potencies, not only growth of leaves were stunted but also they became whitish.

Disease symptoms produced in plants with homoeopathic potencies		
Treatment	6c ptency	1M potency
Kali sulph	Tipsof lower leaes turned yellowish	Lower leaves discoloured as if scorched
Mag sulph	Growth stimulated with bright green leaves	General yellowfing of leaves. Interveinal chlorosis
Zinc sulph	Normal growth with green leaves	Yellow spotting on lower leaf
Cuprum sulph	Growth stunted. Tips of leaves pale and inclined to die	Growth stunted. Tip of leaves dead and ddecolorized
Ferrum sulph	Leaf colour light yellow, with stunted growth	Leaf colour whitish with remarkable stunted growth
Control : Leaf colour comparatively dull and less vigorous		

Figure 13.1

The toxicity symptoms thus produced were found to be more developed with 1M (one thousand centesimal) potency than with the 6c potency.

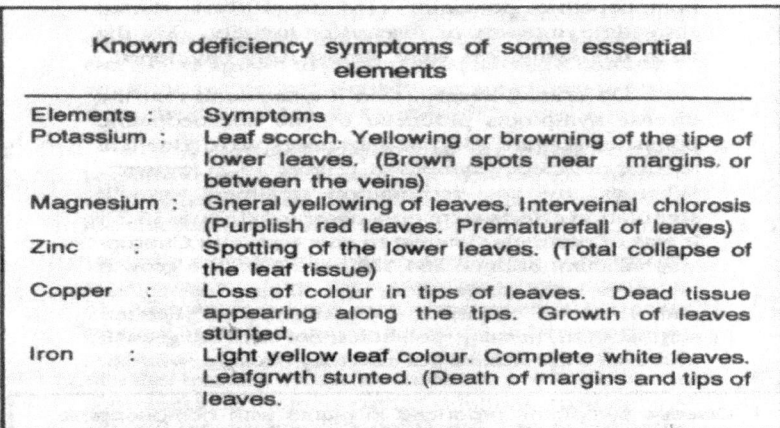

Figure 13.2

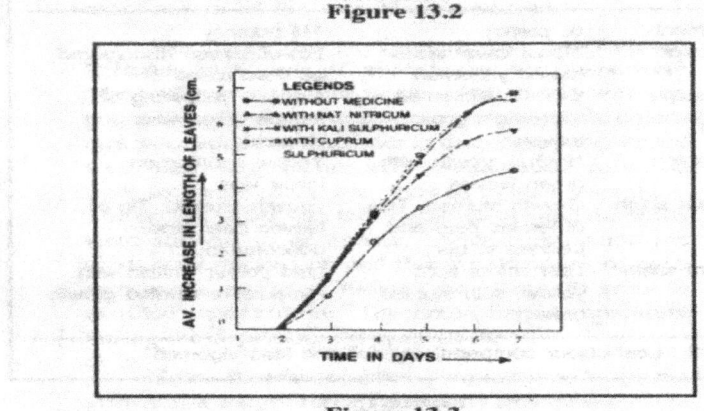

Figure 13.3

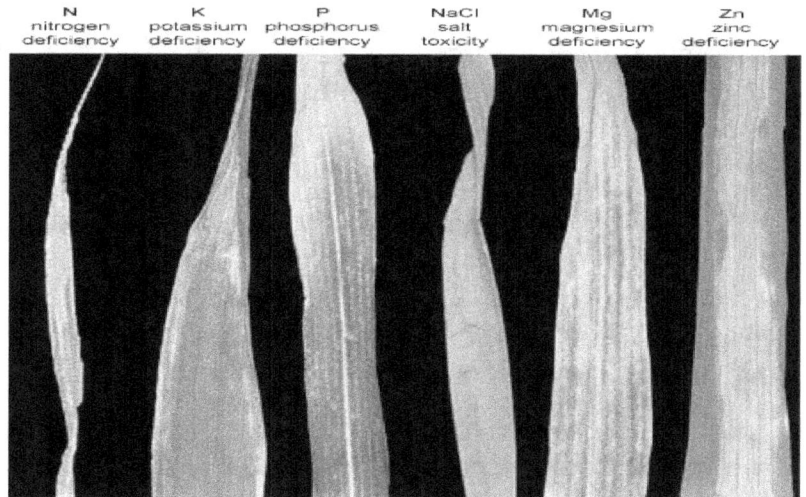

Figure 13.4

On the basic of the above observations it could be inferred that the specific disease symptoms in plants are cured by the essential elements not because the diseases were caused due to deficiency of the elements, but because similar diseases symptoms can be produced by the same elements in toxic level.

In this connection it may be further noted that although there is no reliable evidence of plants producing antibodies yet different kinds of disease resistance in plants are known, notably an induced resistance, that is analogous to be antigen-antibody immunological system of animals including humans[67].

Most of the micro-nutrients are also known to be associated with 'enzyme' system of plants[65] and while immune response to various antigens is said to be under controlling influence of genes termed as immune response (Ir) genes, many of the effects of genes are believed to be carried out by enzymes[68].

Not only the colour and character of leaf, shoot, fruit etc. are governed by genes but also the chemical composition of plant tissues are known to be controlled genetically. The greenness of plant is due to certain genes that govern the synthesis of green pigment[69].

A change in genetic make-up termed as 'mutation' is known to affect the normal expression of a gene or a set of genes. No spontaneous mutation has, however, been identified in wheat and rice, which can only be induced by using certain chemical and physical agents[69,70].

Retention of the molecular properties of the substances at high homoeopathic dilutions (potencies) far beyond the negative exponent of Avogadro's number and also their further intensification with the degree of dynamisation is indicative of the existence of light isotopic molecules being formed in the process of homoeopathic potentization, as has been postulated earlier[13].

In recent times the main line of defense against many plant diseases is the development of immune or resistant varieties of the host plants, either by exposing to infection or artificial crossing (hybridization) of parents of known characteristics. An alternative to sexual method of plant improvement is to manipulate plant systems at the cellular level, by artificial fusion of parent cells in tissue culture[70].

Induction of variations in the cell by treating with mutagenic agents is also a modern method. The most speculative method, however, seems to be 'gene-manipulation', wherein nitrogen fixing gene of micro-organism or blue-green algae is contemplated to be transferred to higher plants [70,71]. Success of such a method is of course yet to be seen.

Meanwhile the homoeopathic system of treatment may be effectively and satisfactorily applied in agriculture, to fight out plant diseases through artificial stimulation of immune response in plants. This will not only be economic compared to the existing systems of treatment but also convenient being based on the symptoms, the total modifications shown in plants as a result of the disease, while determination of the causal agent is said to be difficult and usually involves considerable expense of time and labour.

14. The Fate of Homeopathy in the Scientific World of 21st Century

In about 1910, T.H. Morgan, the Nobel laureate, observed that attempts were being made to identify certain gross physical human types, such as bilious, lymphatic, nervous etc. Some of these were supposed to be more susceptible to certain ailments or diseases than the other types, which in turn have their own constitutional characteristics. These well intended efforts were, however, so far in advance of our genetic information that the geneticists may be excused if they refuse to discuss them seriously[72].

Today it has been known that many of the metabolic disorders are due to some defects at the genetic level. In chronic diseases of adult life, a genetic element is particularly believed to be present[16]. More than 1600 human diseases are known to be caused by defects in the contents or the expression of the genetic information in DNA molecules[73].

A probable way to rectify such genetic defects is to replace or supplement the defective gene with a new healthy gene, a process called, 'gene therapy'[74]. But the isolation of the substitute gene in fairly large number and also the methodology of introducing such genes into the defective cells are among many of the formidable problems, which are to be solved before the contemplated 'gene therapy' can be successfully carried out.

For instance, in a diabetic patient, one of the genes involved in insulin production may be defective in the pancreas, which is to be replaced by a substitute gene. This necessitates the introduction of the gene to the specific site i.e. into the particular tissue. Moreover, the same tissue may consist of a few billion cells, most of them being defective, replacement of them may be an arduous task. Further, even if all these are possible in some future date, there is again no guarantee that the substitute genes will behave according to the command of the host cell[74].

On the other hand, in case of 'genetic engineering' the basic tools are enzymes known as 'restriction endonucleases', which cleave DNA chains at specific sequences, because of the way the chains are snipped, the so-called 'sticky ends' can join together again or with sticky ends of foreign DNA that has been cut by the same enzyme. The new plasmid (circular genetic element residing in the cell cytoplasm of some bacteria) is referred to as a 'recombinant DNA'. The next step is to insert the hybrid plasmid back into the host, where after it will be theoretically treated as normal DNA.

Among the proposed benefits of the technique are the constructions of bacteria capable of producing insulin and also engineering of plants that can manufacture their own nitrogen compounds[75]. Further, spectacular applications of genetic engineering are being contemplated, with fabrication of DNA sequences by chemical synthesis on the one hand, and by using the recombinant DNA technology on the other hand, to clone it and make unlimited amounts and then insert to any piece of DNA according to choice. Thus a new research activity has been directed towards 'controlled mutation', as has been termed by Khorana[76].

It is, however, generally believed that in the foreseeable future the genetic engineering will be primarily use for exploring the ways the genes are controlled in man, rather than allowing man to control his genes[76]. Some scientists are also worried that in cutting up the genetic material of higher organisms, recombinant DNA researchers may accidentally include undesirable piece of DNA in the hybrid plasmids. Bacteria containing such plasmids would then be uniquely pathogenic and may cause hazard to human lives. Restrictions of DNA recombinant researches have, therefore, been imposed in various countries[77].

Thus while at the moment the scientific world seems to be rather lost in the glamorous and clamorous event occurring in the fields of genetic engineering as well as gene-therapy, 'homoeopathy', the only possible from of 'genetic treatment', is lying discarded and disregarded. The claim that the permanent genetic defects (mutations) may be corrected through a process of 'reverse mutation' triggered by the quantum of action of the high energy light isotopic particles, contained in the homoeopathic potencies, is yet to receive a scientific recognition and acceptance.

Hahnemann is said to have been born before his time. So his theories of 'similia similibus curentur' and 'chronic miasm', met with the same fate as that of many other discoveries which were made ahead on their time. Their significances were not realized and they feel into oblivion even the countries of their origin.

But then, Gregor Mendel was given the recognition, as the father of 'genetics' only in early 20th century, many years after his death. Avogadro's hypothesis was resurrected fifty years after its first publication and took about equal time thereafter for its final acceptance. Various observations for Hahnemann made in early nineteenth century, got scientific footings in late twentieth century, due to spectacular discoveries made in various fields of micro-sciences.

It is, therefore, evident that new waves of progress will descend soon in this 21st Century, making thereby the universal acceptance of homoeopathy as unavoidable.

15. HOMOEOPATHIC ANTIBIOTICS??

Homoeopathic Antibiotics? I am sure this term itself is sufficient to infuriate the so called 'Classical Homoeopaths' and even those who don't claim to be such ardent followers of our Great Master (Dr Samuel Hahnemann) would also raise a brow about it.

Like it or not but believe me this is a reality, of course if you consider mother tinctures to be Homoeopathic drugs. If Crataegus Q, Passiflora Q, Alfalfa Q OR Hydrastis Q can find a place in the prescriptions of most Homoeopaths, why not another 56 herbs which can safely be called 'Homoeopathic Antibiotics'.

In a recent study done by the department of Agricultural Microbiology, Institute of Agriculture, Aligarh Muslim University, total of 82 Indian Medicinal Plants traditionally used in medicines were subjected to preliminary ANTIBACTERIAL SCREENING against several Pathogenic and opportunistic Micro-organisms.

Aqueous, hexane and alcoholic extracts of each plant was tested for their antibacterial activity using Agar well diffusion method at sample concentration of 200mg /ml. The result showed that out of 82 plants under screening, 56 exhibited antibacterial activity against one or more test pathogens.Amazingly extracts of 5 plants showed strong and Broad spectrum activity as compared to rest of 51 plant extracts which demonstrated moderate activity.On the whole, the alcoholic extracts showed greater activity than their corresponding aqueous and hexane extracts. Among various extracts , only alcoholic extracts of Embelica officinalis, Terminalia Chebula, Terminalia

Belerica, Plumbago zeylanica and Holarrhena antidysenterica were found to show potentially interesting activity against test Bacteria. These crude alcoholic extracts were also assayed for cellular toxicity to fresh sheep erythrocytes and found to have no cellular toxicity.

In another study undertaken by the Institute of Pharmacognosy, University of Gras, Australia, Holarrhena antidysenterica stem bark was tested for antibacterial efficacy against Staphylococcus aureus, Staphylococcus epidermidis, Streptococcus faecalis, Bacillus subtilis, Eschiricia coli and Pseudomonas aeruginosa using the microdilution broth method as well as disc diffusion , method. The crude methanolic extract was active against all tested Bacteria.Further a chemical fractionation indicated that the antibacterial activity was mainly associated with the alkaloids. The minimum inhibitory concentration (MIC) and Minimum Bactericidal Concentration (MBC) were determined for the crude extracts , the total alkaloids and the neutral fraction using Microdilution broth method. The results were compared with other reputed antibiotics.The total alkaloids showed remarkable ac tivity against Staphylococcus aureus(MIC =95 microgram / ml).

PHYTOCHEMICAL ANALYSIS OF HOLARRHENA ANTIDYSENTERICA

Around 30 alkaloids have been isolated from the plant, mostly from the bark. These include conessine, kurchine, kurchicine, holarrhimine, conarrhimine, conaine, conessimine, iso-conessimine, conimine, holacetin and conkurchin

Pharmacology of H.Antidysenterica

Conessine from the bark killed free living amoebae and also kills entamoeba histolytica in the dysenteric stools of experimentally infected kittens. It is markedly lethal to the flagellate protozoon. It is antitubercular also.

Microbiological Profile of Kurchi(H.Antidysenterica) Extract(Table A)

Total bacterial count	Not more than 3000 CFU/gm
Yeasts and moulds	Not more than 100 CFU/gm
E.coli	Absent
S.aureus	Absent
Salmonella typhi	Absent
Pseudomonas aeruginose	Absent

(Table A)

PHYTOCHEMICAL ANALYSIS OF TERMINALIA CHEBULA

Chemical composition: Fruits contain astringent substances - tannic acid, Chebulinic acid, gallic acid etc. Resin and a purgative principle of the nature of anthraquinone and sennoside are also present.

Pharmacology: Fruit contains a constituent which has a wide antibacterial and antifungal spectrum, and also inhibits growth of E.coli, the most common organism responsible for urinary tract infection.

Microbiological Profile of Terminalia chebula (Table B)

Total bacterial count	Not more than 3000 CFU/gm
Yeasts and moulds	Not more than 100 CFU/gm
E.coli	Absent
S.aureus	Absent
Salmonella typhi	Absent
Pseudomonas aeruginose	Absent

Table B

Antibacterial activity of black Myrobalan (Terminalia chebula Retz) against Helicobacter pylori(Research by Department of Microbiology and Biological Sciences, University of Tehran, Tehran, Iran; Center of Marine Biotechnology, Biotechnology Institute, University of Maryland USA; Department of Cell and Molecular Genetics, University of Maryland, USA)

The effect of ether, alcoholic and water extracts of black myrobalan (Teminalia chebula Retz) on Helicobactor pylori were examined using an agar diffusion method on Columbia Agar. Water extracts of black myrobalan showed significant antibacterial activity and had a minimum inhibitory concentration (MIC) and minimum bacteriocidal concentration (MBC) of 125 and 150 mg/l, respectively. The extract was active after autoclaving for 30 min at 121°C. Plant powder (incorporated in agar) gave higher MIC and MBC values (150 and 175 mg/l, respectively). Water extracts of the black myrobalan at a concentration of 1-2.5 mg/ml inhibited urease activity of H. pylori. The results show that black myrobalan extracts contain a heat stable agent(s) with possible therapeutic potential. Other bacterial species were also inhibited by black myrobalan water extracts.

Influenced by these findings, I, conducted a research to identify the antibiotic properties of Terminali Chebula and Holarrhena antidysenterica mother tinctures on two groups of Bacteria , E-Coli and Staphylococcus aureus.

In Vitro Action of Holarrhena Antidysenterica(Kurchi) Q and Terminalia chebula Q on E-coli and Staphylococcus aureus.

Collection of Sample: Early Morning Mid-stream Urine(30 ml) was collected in a sterile Test Tube, from a female patient diagnosed to be suffering from Urinary Tract Infection(UTI).

APPLICATION OF MEDICINES

The sample was divided into 10 sterile Test Tubes(1 ml in each tube), and the following drugs were applied(Table1):

Test Tube	Content(Added to sample)
Test Tube 1	Sample + Distilled water
Test Tube 2	Sample + Rectified Spirit
Test Tube 3	Sample + Kurchi Q
Test Tube 4	Sample + Terminalia chebula Q
Test Tube 5	Sample + Kurchi 30
Test Tube 6	Sample + Terminalia chebula 30
Test Tube 7	Sample + Kurchi 200
Test Tube 8	Sample + Terminalia chebula 200
Test Tube 9	Sample + Kurchi 1M
Test Tube 10	Sample + Terminalia chebula 1M

Table 1

The Test tubes were left alone for 2 hours and the contents were allowed to act.

PREPARATION OF CULTURE MEDIA

For Quantitative analysis of Bacteria Colony, plate culture of Molten agar was prepared in 10 sterile petri dishes and 1 ml of the contents of the 10 test tubes were poured into it and allowed to set.

0.5 ml of distilled water, rectified spirit, and the medicines were added again in these petri dishes in serial order. This set up was incubated at 37 degree centigrade for 24 Hours.

The result of colony count after Gram staining reveals the following(Table 2):

Test Tube	Drugs Applied	No. Of Bacteria per High power field
TT1	Distilled Water	10-12
TT2	Rectified Spirit	11-13
TT3	Kurchi Q	6-7
TT4	Terminalia chebula Q	7-8
TT5	Kurchi 30	11-12
TT6	Terminalia chebula 30	11-12
TT7	Kurchi 200	11-12
TT8	Terminalia chebula 200	11-12
TT9	Kurchi 1M	11-12
TT10	Terminalia chebula 1M	11-12

Table 2

CULTURE IN NUTRIENT BROTH MEDIA

To 6 sterile Petri Dishes, containing Nutrient Broth Media,1 ml of Urine sample(collected previously was added).

Water, Rectified Spirit, Mother Tinctures and Potentised medicines was added to them in serial order, incubation for 24 hours gave the following result(Table 3):

Petri Dish	Medicines Added(0.5 ml)	Turbidity
PD1	Distilled Water	+++
PD2	Rectified Spirit	+++
PD3	Kurchi Q	+
PD4	Terminalia Chebula Q	++
PD5	Kurchi 30	+++
PD6	Terminalia Chebula 30	+++
PD7	Kurchi 200	+++
PD8	Terminalia Chebula 200	+++
PD9	Kurchi 1M	+++
PD10	Terminalia Chebula 1M	+++

Table 3

Similar results were also obtained in MacConkey's media where samples were treated with Kurchi Q and Terminalia Chebula Q,showed 'NO Change' while others turned Pink in colour.

Inference

These findings clearly demonstrate that Holarrhena antidysenterica Q and Terminalia Chebula Q are Bacteriostatic on E.Coli. The higher potencies of these two drugs are however seen to possess no such direct Bacteriostatic property.

ACTION OF HOMOEOPATHIC MOTHER TINCTURES ON STAPHYLOCOCCUS AUREUS

Samples of pus from suppurative skin lesion was collected in a sterile and observed under microscope after Gram staining. Gram Positive cocci(Round shaped Bacteria) arranged in grape like clusters, suggested the presence of Staphylococcus.

The sample of pus was then divided into 6 equal parts (1 ml each) after diluting it with normal saline solution.

These 6 parts were then transferred to 6 sterile petri dishes and was treated with distilled water, Rectified spirit , H.antidysenterica Q, Terminalia chebula Q, H.antidysenterica 200 and Terminalia chebula 200 in serial order.

Six sets of Nutrient Agar media were prepared and 1%Glycol monoacetate was added to it to enhance pigment production. The samples were then transferred to the culture media in serial order. Application

Of all the medicines along with the control fluids were repeated once more by inoculation method.

After incubation of 24 hours , at 37 degree centigrade, the pattern given below was observed(Table 4):

Petri Dish	Medicines Added	Colony Type	Colony Diameter
PD1	Distilled Water	Circular, Convex, Smooth, Shiny, Opaque, Golden Yellow colonies, were seen.	2-4 mm
PD2	Rectified Spirit	Circular, Convex, Smooth, Shiny, Opaque, Golden Yellow colonies, were seen.	2-4 mm
PD3	Kurchi Q	No Colony formation seen	-
PD4	Terminalia Chebula Q	A very few colonies were seen, faint Golden yellow in colour.	1 mm in diameter
PD5	Kurchi 30	Golden yellow colonies seen	2-4 mm
PD6	Terminalia Chebula 30	Golden yellow colonies seen	2-4 mm

Table 4

Inference:

Holarrhena antidysenterica Q and Terminalia Chebula Q are Bacteriostatic on Staphylococcus aureus. The higher potencies of these two drugs, are however seen to possess no such direct Bacteriostatic action on this group of Bacterium.

Extensive clinical trials have been conducted with these medicines in cases of UTI and Sore throat and excellent results have been achieved.

While the classical homoeopaths might argue that they have cured several cases of bacterial diseases e.g Typhoid, UTI etc. with potentised medicines, what is the need to opt for such non Homoeopathic measures? I agree, I myself have treated numerous patients by using the higher potencies and firmly believe that potentised homoeopathic medicines alone carry the real essence of

Homoeopathy and are capable to work wonders, but it is also a common phenomenon that many times it seems that the case is going out of hand and there is no way left except referring the patients to Allopathic physicians who in turn administer the patients with harmful antibiotics like Ciprofloxacin, Ofloxacin, etc. The patients get cured but suffers in future from the side effects of these harmful chemicals.

HOMOEOPATHIC ANTIBIOTICS

Homoeopathic antibiotics provide the doctor with one more option to combat with the different micro-organisms in a comparatively safer way. So next time you get a case of E.Coli Urinary tract infection or Staphylococcal sore throat try out Kurchi Q or Terminalia chebula Q tinctures in a dosage of 20 drops thrice daily for two to three days and observe the result.Your successes or failures if sent to me would be of immense value in my research.

Remember the Physician's mission is to cure in the safest way in the quickest possible time.So now you decide, in your next hopeless case, whether to send your patient to an Allopathic physician for another course of strong Antibiotics or just try out these safer Mother tinctures .Publish your results for the benefit of Homoeopathy. There is just one way to take this mode of treatment to newer heights and to make it more convenient and popular amongst the patients and that is only 'RESEARCH work.'

The fear of distorting Homoeopathy can be kept aside for the moment as research not only tells us what to do but also tells us what not to do. Homoeopathic Antibiotics would probably bring the much needed change in Homoeopathic therapy and give homoeopaths the weapon they so desperately wanted in their armory .This Research(First published in 2004 in Homoeopathy for All) will remain as a pioneer work in this field – something done and said which was never done earlier, probably because no one 'Dared to'(be wise).

16. HOMOEOPATHY IN PAIN MANAGEMENT
Pain is inevitable suffering is optional

International Association for the Study of Pain (IASP) as "an unpleasant sensory and emotional experience associated with actual or potential tissue damage, or described in terms of such damage.

In medicine pain is considered highly subjective. Diagnosis is based on characterizing pain in various ways, according to duration, intensity, type (dull, burning, throbbing or stabbing), source, or location in body.

Usually, 'acute' pain stops without treatment or responds to simple measures such as resting or taking an analgesic. Sometimes acute pain may also become intractable and develop into a condition called chronic pain, in which pain is no longer considered a symptom but an illness by itself.

Pain is part of the body's defense mechanism, triggering a reflex reaction to retract or pull away from a painful stimulus, and helps adjust behavior to increase avoidance of that particular harmful situation in the future.

Role of Nociceptors in pain:

Nociception (synonym: nocioception or nociperception) is defined as "the neural processes of encoding and processing noxious stimuli.

Mechanical, thermal, and chemical stimuli are detected by nerve endings called nociceptors, which are found in the skin and on internal surfaces such as the periosteum or joint surfaces. The concentration of nociceptors varies throughout the body, mostly found in the skin and less so in deep internal surfaces. All nociceptors are free nerve endings that have their cell bodies outside the spinal column in the dorsal root ganglia and are named according to their appearance at their sensory ends.

Nociceptors have a certain threshold; that is, they require a minimum level of stimuli before they trigger a signal. In some conditions, excitation of pain fibers becomes greater as the pain stimulus continues, leading to a condition called hyperalgesia. Once the threshold is reached a signal is passed along the axon of the nerve into the spinal cord.

Mechanism

Stimulation of a nociceptor, due to a chemical, thermal, or mechanical cause that has the potential to damage body tissue, may cause **nociceptive pain**.

Damage to the nervous system itself, due to disease or trauma, may cause **neuropathic** (or neurogenic) pain. Neuropathic pain may refer to peripheral neuropathic pain, which is caused by damage to nerves, or to central neuropathic pain, which is caused by damage to the brain, brainstem, or spinal cord.

Nociceptive pain and neuropathic pain are the two main kinds of pain when the primary mechanism of production is considered. A third kind may be mentioned: **psychogenic pain**. Psychogenic pain sufferers are often stigmatized, because both medical professionals and the general public tend to think that pain from a psychological source is not "real". However, specialists consider that it is no less actual or hurtful than pain from other sources.

Pain management

Pain being recognized as a disease in itself, has given rise to different methods of treatment. Patients are willing to spend any amount of money to get relief from pain. In some cases it has been observed that relief from pain is more important to the patient than relief from the causative disease itself e.g Cancer pain, Arthritic pain etc.

Medical management of pain has given rise to a distinction between acute pain and chronic pain.

In general, physicians are more comfortable treating acute pain, which usually is caused by soft tissue damage, infection and/or inflammation among other causes. It is usually treated simultaneously with pharmaceuticals, commonly analgesics, or appropriate techniques for removing the cause and for controlling the pain sensation. The failure to treat acute pain properly may lead to chronic pain in some cases.

Often, patients suffering from chronic pain are referred to various medical specialists. Multidisciplinary pain clinics have been growing in number over the last few decades.

Few methods to treat pain are:

1) **Anesthesia**: is the condition of having the feeling of pain and other sensations blocked by drugs that induces a lack of awareness.

2) **Analgesia**: is an alteration of the sense of pain without loss of consciousness. The body possesses an endogenous analgesia system, which can be supplemented with painkillers or analgesic drugs to regulate nociception and pain.

3) **Traditional Chinese medicine** views pain as a 'blocked' qi(energy flow), akin to electrical resistance, with treatments such as acupuncture claimed as more effective for no traumatic pain than traumatic pain. Although the mechanism is not fully understood, acupuncture may stimulate the release of large quantities of endogenous opioids.

4) **Use of nutritional supplements**: curcumin, glucosamine, chondroitin, bromelain and omega-3 fatty acids. There is interest in the relationship between vitamin D and pain, but the evidence of its relationship to pain other than osteomalacia from controlled trials appears unconvincing.

5) **Hypnosis** as well as diverse perceptional techniques provoking altered states of consciousness have proven to be of important help in the management of all types of pain

Interventional pain management: is the discipline of medicine devoted to the diagnosis and treatment of pain related disorders principally with the application of interventional techniques in managing sub acute, chronic, persistent, and intractable pain, independently or in conjunction with other modalities of treatment. It recognizes different 'Pain Circuits' and treat pain by blocking these pain circuits.

1.Epidural Steroid Injection (Lumbar, Cervical and Thoracic)-it is a process that injects a small amount of powerful anti-inflammatory medication like cortisone around spinal nerves in the epidural space. ESI is used to treat pain caused by inflammation of the spine that may involve herniated discs, pinched nerves, and injured soft and connective tissues. This is almost similar to labor epidurals except that labor epidurals use anaesthetics instead of cortisone (which is an anti inflammatory drug).

2. **Selective nerve root Block**-Spinal nerve compression whether due to disc protrusion or bony canal narrowing can produce symptoms of pain, numbness and weakness. Collateral nerve innervation, referral pain and anatomical variations however can make diagnosis of specific nerve compression difficult especially when patients present with indistinct symptoms.

3. **Facet Medial Branch Block (Lumbar, Cervical and Thoracis** Facet joints are the paired joints that connect vertebrae in the spine. They are important for both range of motion and stability. Over time and with physical stress these joints can erode, enlarge and become arthritic. Facet Medial Branches are the small branches of spinal nerves that innervate these joints. Facet medial branch blocks help to reduce pain from joints and muscles and facilitate physical rehabilitation.

4. Facet Medial Branch Radiofrequency Thermocoagulation - RFTC :*Radiofrequency ablation* or *lesioning* is a treatment by using radiowaves and heat to destroy tissue or a nerve, for pain relief. Radiofrequency has also been used for treating fast heartbeats and tumors with great success.

• Other methods of intervention pain management include:Discography, **Sympathetic Block (Stellate ganglion and Lumbar Sympathetic Blocks), Radiofrequency Lesioning**(Nerves are desensitized by using specialized radiofrequency needles for longer lasting effect than what is achieved with local anesthetics.),**Cryoanalgesia**(Ice being one of the oldest form of pain treatment, Cryoanalgesia uses specialized machine and needle to render nerves insensitive to pain), **Percutaneous Disc Decompression, Intrathecal Pumps (Morphine Pump), Stellate Ganglion Block, Lumbar Sympathetic Block, Celiac Plexus Block, Spinal Cord Stimulator, Sacroiliac Join Injections, Trigger Point Injections etc.**

Homoeopathic pain management:

Homoeopathic pain management remedies not only offer relief from temporary pain disorders but can ensure long term healing as well.

I will discuss the modus operandi of Homoeopathic medicines in pain management in a separate article, however, I would like to point out a few interesting observations:

Minerals, being one of the 6 major sources of Homoeopathic Medicine, play an important role in pain management. **Zinc and copper** may help in wound healing and reduce pain and inflammation (Honkanen, 1991, Lansdown, 1996). **Magnesium** is analgesic for neuropathic pain in animal studies (Begon, 2002) and has shown clinical benefit in the treatment of migraine, cluster and tension headaches (Peikert, 1996; Mauskop, 1996; Demirkaya, 2001). It is unclear whether magnesium can reduce pain related to surgery (Hoinig, 1998; Ko, 2001). Magnesium's mechanism of action in pain management may be partly due to NMDA blockade (Begon, 2002).

Enzymes are substances that influence chemical reactions. Bromelain, a complex enzyme of pineapple, is commonly used in Europe as an anti-inflammatory compound for many forms of musculoskeletal injury, arthritis, cramps, post-surgery and post-traumatic swelling. It has been shown to be beneficial in reducing swelling, inflammation and pain by blocking the creation of proinflammatory compounds like prostaglandins, decreasing the production of kinins, and inhibiting fibrin production (Tasman, 1964). Although it is generally well tolerated, it can aggravate ulcers or esophagitis, and can interact with blood thinners (Meletis, 2000).

Homoeopathic medicines, in Dynamized form , contain light isotopes of the Drug substance(Homoeopathy in the Light of Modern Science – Dr.A.C.Dutta B Jain Publishers). Plant experiments with high Homoeopathic potencies, beyond the negative exponent of Avogadro's number, indicate that the bio chemical effects of the substances are still retained. In the process of homoeopathic potentization, specific positronium complexes are formed, which due to their micro-isotope like behavior, retain the properties of the original molecules, even when they no longer exist.

Light isotopes owing to their very small size penetrates to the level of the genes to correct mutations(as most diseases today are known to be an effect of genetic mutations or anomalies).This process is called Reverse Mutation and resembles 'Hering's law of cure' almost exactly(diseases get cured in the reverse order of their first coming. **Reverse mutation (reversion)** The production by further mutation of a premutation gene from a mutant gene. This reverse mutation restores the ability of the gene to produce a functional protein. Strictly, reversion is the correction of a mutation (i.e. it occurs at the same site); more loosely, the term is applied also to a mutation at another site that masks or suppresses the effect of the first mutation (in fact such organisms are not non-mutant, but double mutants with the same phenotype).

So, role of Homoeopathic medicine in pain management is two fold: Biochemical analgesic effect and enzyme alteration to block Pain factors.

Patent Medicines: The classical school might still debate the role of combination medicines in Homoeopathy but in Science- Observations cannot be just ruled out. The patent combination medicines in numerous cases have been found to give relief to the patients in cases of pain- both of traumatic and pathological origin.

17. UNIVERSAL SCIENTIFIC RECOGNITION TO HOMOEOPATHY
IS
INEVITABLE

Medical Science vis-a -vis Homoeopathy :

On the well known concept of Hippocrates, the further of Medical Science that – Diseases might be cured either by 'opposites' or 'similars', - Hahnemann through exhaustive experimental observations established homoeopathic system of medicine, on the basis of 'similia similibus curentur'. At the same time he named the conventional medical system based on 'opposites' as Allopathy. Hence Homoeopathy and Allopathy do not posses any controversy among themselves; rather they may be called as, two different branches of the same tree, that is – Medical Science.

So any attempt to ridicule and / or defame homoeopathy, ultimately undermines medical science and also it's Father – Hippocrates.

High Dilution a Paradox:

Unfortunately, almost since its inception a great deal of controversy persist on the question of scientificity of homoeopathy.

Hahnemann's use of insignificantly small doses of medicine was particularly a matter of ridicule from scientific stand point. Initially, intended to get rid of adverse toxic effects of drug substances, Hahnemann made frequent use of greatly diluted medicines, and soon he was convinced of much higher efficacy of such greatly diluted medicines.

Although later on he professed in his work, 'On Chronic Diseases', that it indeed took lot of self-conviction to believe that such an incredibly small medical dose could have an effect for so many weeks. He did not demand that anyone believe him and did not expect this to be conceivable to anyone. He himself could not conceive of it either. But it was fact and experiences confirmed that it was so.

But then, with the resurrection of Avogadro's hypothesis in 1860, it was confirmed that beyond the homoeopathic 12 C dilution, there cannot exist any molecule of the original drug substances.

Further, as per established science matter is not infinitely divisible, and molecules are the ultimate units of transaction in any chemical or bio-chemical reaction. So any dilution of matter to such a stage where hardly a unit of the drug substance is likely to be encountered in a given does of medicine looses all meaning in scientific sense.

Confronted with this awkward situation various propositions and postulations were put forward in support of homoeopathic potentized medicines, mainly based on the vehicle ethanol and / or water, which is carried over from the beginning to the end point. But unfortunately the propositions could not be scientifically acceptable as because the properties of substance are known to depend not on the external orientations and arrangements of the molecules, but on the internal electronic configurations of atoms of the substances.

Revolutionary Role of Scientific Hypothesis:

Hence the course of further advancement and scientific recognition of homoeopathy seems to be stagnated not due to lack of experimental supports but for want of a well demarcated scientific hypothesis, in support of homoeopathic potentized medicine and its mode of action.

Importance of scientific hypothesis is clearly demonstrated by Noble Prize winning examples of Watson and Crick's hypothesis on DNA structure; Jern's hypothesis on the origin of immunological diversity; and Mitchell's hypothesis on oxidative phosphorylation, which incidentally revolutionized the fields concerned.

With advancement of modern science, as well as, some spectacular discoveries in late 20th century, particularly in fields of micro-chemistry, micro-physics and micro-biology, today it has been possible to put forward a well demarcated scientific hypothesis in support of homoeopathic potentized medicine and its mode of action. They hypothesis titled – 'Homoeopathy, a light isotopic mode of genetic treatment' was accepted for presentation in the Indian Science Congress, 1977, New Delhi and was honoured with a special lecture.

Incidentally, the keynote of the hypothesis is found to surprisingly in concordance with **Hahnemann's famous observation made in his 'Lesser Writings (P.734)' as follows – "By means of such trituration and succusion, the internal material power is wonderfully developed and is as it were liberated from its material** bounds, so as to enable it to operate more penetratingly and more freely upon the human organism."

Creation of Ultra – Micro Molecules:

Earlier the notion was matter or mass can neither be created nor destroyed. But today it is known that matter can be created by materialization of a quantum of electromagnetic energy into an electro positron pair or 'positronium unit' of ultra – micro from of elementary particles to a pair of gamma rays. Pair production is of considerable theoretical interest in particle science, as a striking confirmation of the relativistic quantum theory proposed by Dirac.

Due to similar single electronic configuration and at the same time infinitesimal mass, the positronium units are said to behave like – isotope of hydrogen. Existence of two such isotopes, i.e. light – isotopes of Helium and Lithium have also been confirmed scientifically through indirect evidences. Because direct observation of a particles of such small mass is difficult due to considerable Doppler broadening caused of thermal energies.

Hence, in the process of homoeopathic potentization, the light isotopes of the drug substances are created due to some unforeseeable factors. Such as first of all high electrostatic charges are developed during succusion due to friction between the ethanol molecules and the glass vials. Incidentally ethanol molecules are known posses high 'electron affinity'. Subsequently, in the strong electric fields thus produced, through absorption of electro – magnetic waves 'electron – position pairs' or 'positronium units' are created spontaneously.

Thereafter, the positronium units thus created in the surroundings of the 'polar' molecules of ethanol are not only supposed to be more stable but also induced by the specific molecules fields of the microscopic drug particles, which are also known to behave like mini – magnets – specifically clump together to give birth to light – isotopes of the drug substances, in increasing concentrations due auto – catalytic effect.

Thus even when the conventional macro – molecules of the drug substances are eliminated due to serial dilution, the therapeutic properties of the medicinal substances are retained more powerfully and more penetratingly through the ultra – micro light – isotopic drug particles created in the process of homoeopathic potentization. **This is very much in concordance with the first part of Hahnemann's observation as follows – "By means of such trituration and succussion the internal medicinal power is wonderfully developed and is as it were liberated from its material bonds,…"**

Genetic Drug Effects of Homoeopathic Potencies :

Today is has been known that many of the metabolic disorders are due to some / functional and / or structural defects in the genetic level. More than 1600 human diseases are said to be caused by defects in the contents or the expression of genetic information, encoded in the DNA molecules.

Further, as per some recent observation, any agent in its ultra – microscopic from that can penetrate to the chromosome level, having localized chemical effects can exert it's influences into the genetic information.

Hence in acute diseases, homoeopathic potentized medicines functioning like 'antigens', stimulate the body's specific antigen – antibody like immunological response under the controlling influence of immune response (Ir) genes, thereby cure the disease conditions, overcoming the functional genetic defects.

Whereas in case of chronic diseases, developed due to structural genetic defect, called 'gene mutation' – homoeopathic potentized medicines functioning like 'anti-mutagen's i.e. in classical homoeopathic term 'anti-misam's, trigger the body's specific 'reverse mutation' process, when symptoms reappear in the reverse order of their first coming until the chronic disease condition is fully cured.

Thus the second part of Hahnemann's observation is also amply enlightened as follows –

" so as to enable it to operate more penetratingly and more freely upon human organism."

Established Science was lagging Behind Homoeopathy:

For nearly two hundred years homoeopathy remained scientifically inconceivable. This is because the established science was lagging behind and hence Hahnemann was said to have come much ahead of his time. But then, by late twentieth century, due to some spectacular discoveries and advancement in micro-sciences and quantum mechanics, today homoeopathy has got solid scientific footing and emerging as – the ultra – micro medicinal system for the new millennium.

18. HOMOEOPATHY A LIGHT ISOTOPIC MODE OF GENTIC TREATMENT.

Medical Science vis –a – vis Homoeopathy:

On the well known concept of Hippocrates, the Father of Medical Science that – Diseases might be cured either by 'opposites' or 'similars', -Hahnemann through exhaustive experimental observations established Homoeopathic System of treatment on the basis of 'similars' i.e. 'Similia Similibus Curentur'.At the same time he named the conventional medicinal system based on 'opposites' as Allopathy. Hence Homoeopathy and Allopathy do not posses any controversy among themselves. Rather they may be called as two different branches of the same tree, that is - Medical Science.

High Dilution a Paradox:

Unfortunately, almost since its inception a great deal of controversy persists on the question of scientificity of Homoeopathy. Hahnemann's use of insignificantly small doses of medicines was particularly a matter of ridicule from Scientific Stand Point.

Further, as per established science, matter is not infinitely divisible, and 'molecules' are the ultimate units of transaction in any chemical or bio-chemical reaction. So any dilution of matter to such a stage where hardly a unit of the drug substance is likely to be encountered in a given does of medicine loses all meaning in scientific sense.

Confronted with this awkward situation, various propositions and postulations were put forward in support of homoeopathic potentized medicines, mainly based on the vehicle ethanol and / or water, which are carried over from the beginning to the end point. But unfortunately properties of substances are known to depend not on the external arrangement and orientation of the molecules of the vehicles, but on the internal electronic configurations of the atoms of the substances.

Creation of Ultra – Micro Molecules:

Earlier the notion was matter or mass can neither be created nor destroyed. But today it is known that matter can be created by materialization of an electromagnetic energy into an electron positron pair i.e. positronium unit of ultra – micro form. Pair production is of considerable theoretical interest in particle science, as a striking confirmation of relativistic quantum theory proposed by Dirac.

Due to similar single electronic configuration and at the same time infinitesimal mass, due to replacement of 'proton' by 'positron', the positronium units are said to behave like light – isotope of 'hydrogen'. Existence of two more such light – isotopes i.e. of 'Helium' and 'Lithium' have also been confirmed scientifically through indirect evidences. Because direct observation of particles of such small mass is difficult due to considerable Doppler broadening caused at thermal energy.

Hence, in the process of homoeopathic potentization, the light isotopes of the drug substances are created due to some unforeseeable scientific facts. Such as, firstly, development of high electro – static charges due to friction between the 'ethanol' molecules and the 'glass' vial. Subsequently, through absorption of the electro – magnetic waves, positron pairs or 'positronium' units are created spontaneously.

Thereafter, the 'positronium' units thus created in the surrounding of the 'polar' molecules of ethanol, are not only supposed to be more stable but also induced by the specific molecular fields of the microscopic drug particles, which are also known to behave like mini – magnets, they specifically clump together to give birth to the light – isotopes of the drug substances, in increasing concentrations due to their auto – catalytic effects.

Genetic Drug Effects of Homoeopathy Potencies:

Thus even when the conventional macro – molecules of the drug substances are eliminated out due to serial dilution, the therapeutic properties of the medicinal substances are retained more powerfully and more penetratingly through the ultra–micro light–isotopic drug particles created in the process of homoeopathic potentization.

Further, today it has been known the many of the metabolic disorders are caused due to some functional and / or structural defects in the genetic level. More than 1600 human diseases are said to be caused by defects in the contents of expression of genetic information encoded in the DNA molecules.

As per observation, further it has been known that any agent in its ultra – microscopic from, that can penetrate to the chromosome level, having localized chemical effect, can expert its positive influences into the genetic information.

Hence in 'Acute Diseases', Homoeopathic potentized medicines functioning like 'antigens', stimulate the body's specific antigen – antibody like immunological response under the controlling influence of Immune response (Ir)genes, thereby cure the disease conditions, overcoming the 'functional' genetic defects.

Whereas in cases of 'Choric Diseases', developed due to structural genetic defects, called 'gene – mutation's – homoeopathic potentized medicines functioning like 'anti – mutagens' i.e. in classical homoeopathic term 'anti – miasms', trigger the body's specific reverse mutation process, when symptoms reappear in the reverse order of their first coming, until the Chronic disease condition is fully cured.

Scientific Hypothesis vis-à-vis Hahnemann's observation:

Hence the course of further advancement and scientific recognition of homoeopathy seems to be stagnated not due to lack of experimental support but for want of a well demarcated scientific hypothesis, in support of homoeopathic potentized medicines and its mode of action.

Importance of scientific hypothesis is clearly demonstrated by Nobel Prize Winning examples of Watson and Crick's hypothesis on DNA structure; Jern's hypothesis on the origin of immunological diversity and Mitchell's hypothesis on oxidative phosphorylation, which incidentally revolutionized the fields concern.+

Homoeopathy in the Light of Modern Science

With the advancement of modern science as well as, some spectacular discoveries in late 20th Century, particularly in the fields of micro – chemistry, micro – physics and micro – biology, today it has been possible to put forward a well demarcated scientific hypothesis in support of homoeopathic potentized medicine and its mode of action. The scientific hypothesis titled – "Homoeopathy a light isotopic mode of genetic treatment", - was accepted for presentation at the India

Science Congress, 1977, New Delhi, as a special lecture.

Incidentally, the keynote content of the hypothesis is found to be surprisingly in concordance with

Hahnemann's famous observation made in his ' Lesser Writings (P734)' as follows – **"By means of such trituration and succession, the internal medicinal power is wonderfully developed and is it were liberated from its material bonds , so as to enable it to operate more penetratingly and more freely upon the human organism".**

Further, incidentally patronized by Dr. Diwan Harish Chand, President of Honour LMHI, endowed the author with the prestigious Dr. Susil Kumar and Jamila Mitra award 1996, at the hand of Hon'ble Minister of health and family Welfare, Delhi NCR Dr. Harsh Vardhan (Presently the Vice President of CSIR – Council for Scientific and Industrial Research) for discovering the missing link between homoeopathy and modern science.

So the ball is in the court of the World Scientific Community. Now it is upon them whether they should come forward for a universal scientific recognition to Homoeopathy for the benefit of the ailing humanity or turn away faces and remain indifferent.

19. FREQUENTLY ASKED QUESTIONS:-

So before concluding, in view of the above perspective let us deal with some controversial questions as follows:

Q.1) Even if not directly observable, is there any indirect evidence, that the light isotopes of the drug substance are created?

Ans: Yes. Substances like common salt, sand, alumina etc. having practically no medicinal value in crude forms, are known to develop some kind of toxicity in the process of potentisation, achieving thereby extraordinary medicinal power in their Homoeopathic potencies. This may be ascribed only to the creation of their light isotopic forms because isotopes, though having similar chemical properties, are often known to act biochemically at different rates due to their differences in activation energy. Thus water, possessing no toxic effect for any life process, its isotopic form i.e. 'heavy water' is regarded upto a poison.

Q.2) **Is there any evidence that some form of autocatalytic reaction occurs in the process of potentisation?**

Ans) Yes. A peculiar 'On' and 'off 'effect with the homoeopathic potencies, giving a wave like curve as observed by Nebel, Boyd, Benveniste and others can only be ascribed to an auto catalytic effect generated in the process of potentisation. This is because an auto catalytic effect n a liquid phase is graphically expressed by the curve of sine type. Hence, the peak points of the curve such as 6C, 12C, 30C, 200 C etc. are commonly used.

Homoeopathy in the Light of Modern Science

Q3) Homoeopathic potentised medicines are said to be less heat stable. Is it true?

Ans. Yes. This is because the structure of substances on the molecular scale is known to be determined by a balance between the ordering influence of intermolecular forces and disordering influence of the thermal motion. In the homoeopathic potencies the positronium units are supposed to be specifically clumped together by comparatively weak electromagnetic force, due to absence of protons and neutrons. Hence they are less heat stable. Incidentally the wooden chest, glass vessels, velvet cork, paper packs etc. all known as highly resistive to heat.

Q.4) It is said that during the process of potentization the homoeopathic medicines should not be touched with hand, because in that case the medicinal power is said to be not developed. Is it true?

Ans.) Yes. In that case the electro-static charges developed as primary requirement, for development of medicinal power, will be conducted out through the body. Incidentally the glass vessel, velvet corks, porcelain mortar pestles, ebonite spatula etc. all are known to be highly resistive to electricity. Moreover the commercial glass vessels, particularly of straight cylindrical types, are known to be capable of withstanding very high voltage.

Q.5) Is it true that by using water instead of ethanol, and also by not changing the glass vessel at every stage, will lead to the production of poor quality homoeopathic medicines?

Ans. Yes. 'Water' does not possess any strong electron

affinity like that of ethanol molecules, hence the development of electrostatic charges will be extremely poor.

Further, in the process of succussion if at every stage new glass vials and fresh ethanol are taken, the process becomes open and continuous.

Q.6) In the process of potentization is there any specific utility in the stroke method compared to the 'vibration' method?

Ans) Yes. The effect of potentization is not limited to the molecular agitation only, happening during vibration. On the contrary series of unforeseen incidents occur through the stroke method, where the ethanol molecules take a vital role.

Such as due to their strong electron affinity when the ethanol molecules are vigorously flown over the inner surface of the glass vials, strong electro-static charges are produced. Thereafter, due to materialization of electro – magnetic waves 'positronium' units are spontaneously /created, which specifically clump together in the 'polar' environment of ethanol molecules, to give birth to light isotopes of the drug substances.

Further today it has been scientifically established that 'microscopic' particles in suitable environment behave like mini magnets. Thus Hahnemann's analogy of magnetization with that of potentisation appears to be true and also the specific utility of the one way frictional stroke method seems to be quite understandable.

Q.7) Homoeopathy medicines are too slow in acting- is that true?

Ans) This is an Absolutely a wrong conception. Speed of action or recovery of patients depends on (i) Susceptibility of the patient (ii) selection of the medicine and potency and (iii) stage of the disease. If diagnosed early and treated with well selected Homoeopathic medicines, a patient recovers much quicker than Allopathy at times. Unfortunately most patients coming to Homoeopathy after facing failure in other streams of medicines after years of treatment, start expecting magical cure right away – which is impractical. One should remember Homeopathy is no miracle but a medical science and so one who is not ready to undergo a painstaking systematic treatment and rather runs after miracles should not expect a radical cure.

Q.8) Can Homoeopathy and Allopathy be taken together?

Ans) In most cases Homoeopathic medicines can easily be taken along with Allopathic medicines, in fact patients undergoing treatment for some organic diseases like 'Diabetes', 'Thyrotoxicosis', etc are advised not to withdraw the allopathic medicine immediately . In fact in a few cases, a joint therapy is seen to produce better result than both the individual modes of treatment. As Homeopathy acts through the body's natural immune responses , it should not be taken along with those Allopathic medicines that cause Immunosuppression E.g Steroids or Antibiotics

Glossary

Allergen	Pharmacologically active sub-stance.
Antigen	A substance which reacts with the production of specific humoral or cellular immunity
Antibody	A protein found principally in blood serum, originating either normally or in response to an antigen and characterized by a specific reactivity with its com-plimentary antigen.
Antigen- antibody reaction	The combination of an antigen with its antibody.
Astringent	A medicine or other substance that checks discharges of blood, mucus etc
Atom	The smallest particle of an element which can enter into a chemical combination. It is composed of subatomic particles (protons, neutrons, electrons) whose number and arrangement characterize the element.
Avogadro's hypothesis	Under the same conditions of pressure and temperature equal volumes of all gases contain equal number of molecules
Avogadro's number	The number of molecules in a gram molecular weight of a substance is 6.06 x 1CP (cor-rected value being 6.023 x 1CF).
Bacteria	A class of microscopic unicellular or filamentous agents and the cause of many diseases
Basophil	A type of leucocytes that remain coated with IgE (Immunoglobulin E), a protein anti-body.
Carcinogenesis	Production and development of

	cancer.
Catalyst	Catalyst may be gases, liquids and solids. A small amount of catalyst can effect the conver-sion of a large amount of substances — gases, liquids and solids
Catalysts (Auto)	Autocatalytic reactions are a separate class in which one of the reaction products acts catalytically
Compound	A substance whose molecules consist of unlike atoms and whose constituents cannot be separated by physical means.
Complex	A structural whole comprising interconnected parts specially characterized by an involved combination of parts, complicated & intricate. A substance composed of many ingredients.
Contraception	Prevention of conception or impregnation.
Cytotoxic	A substance developed in the blood serum and having a toxic effect upon cells.
Deuterium	Isotope of hydrogen of double mass due to one proton and one neutron (D_2O = Heavy water).
Doppler	Apparent change in the frequency of light or sound ob-served when the source and the observer are in motion relative to one another.
Elementary particle	A particle which in the present state of knowledge cannot be described as compound, and is thus one of the fundamental constituents of a matter Also known as fundamental particle.
Elementary Character	Elementary character of an atom, however, does not change due to excess or deficiency of electron, as

	because this is known to depend on the proton existing in the nucleus of the atom which cannot be easily separated.
Electrostatic	Pertaining to electricity at rest, such as an electric charge on an object.
: Electrostatic	A time-independent electric field, such as that produced by stationary charges.
Electro-magnetic	Pertaining to phenomena in which electricity and magnetism are related
Electro-magnetic field	An electric or magnetic field or a combination of the two, as in an electromagnetic wave
Electro-magnetic wave	A travelling disturbance in space produced by the acceleration of an electric charge, comprising an electric field and a magnetic field at right angles to each other, both moving at the same velocity in a direction normal to the plane of the two fields.
Empirical	Depending on experience or observation alone, without due regard to science and theory.
Enzyme	Any of a class of complex, naturally occurring organic sub-stances of unknown composi-tion that accelerates (catalyze) specific transformation of material in plants and animals.
Etiology	The investigation of the cause of any disease.
Fallow	To plow, harrow and break up a land without seedling for the purpose of destroying weeds and insects and rendering it mellow.
Foliage	Collectively, the mass of leaves or leafage of a plant as produced in nature.

Fusion	The combining of the nuclei or atoms under intense heat to release nuclear energy.
Fusion(Cold)	Same as above under room temperature.
Fission	The splitting of a nucleus of a heavy atom into nuclei of lighter atom and the resultant release of energy.
Fundamental Particles	Any subatomic particle as proton, neutron, electron, nutrino or muon. Quantum theory sug-gested to describe them quanti-tatively.
Gamma rays	Known as electro-magnetic waves similar to visible light (photon particles), but with very short wavelength (invisible), and no change in atomic weight or atomic number is caused by emission of gamma ray.
Gene	A discrete unit (that is each small part) of DNA (deoxyribo-nucleic acid) bound to a protein and arranged linearly in the threadlike structure known as 'chromosome'.
Genetics	The science of heredity etc. pertaining to genes. The unit of chromosome carries and transfers an inherited characteristic from parent to offspring and determines the development of some particular character or trait in the offspring.
Gene mutation	Although generally quite stable, a gene subjected to unusual stress, may undergo a sudden permanent change, known as mutation. A great many substances are known to produce gene mutation Reverse mutations from a mutant to wild type allele is also said to occur
Gene therapy	To replace the defective genes by

	healthy ones
Genetic engineering	Chemical synthesis of DNA sequences, application of DNA recombinant technology by enzyme restriction nucleases, and construction of bacteria with hybrid plasmid.
Gram-molecule	The quantity of a compound or element which has a weight in grams equal numerically to its molecular weight.
Hormone	A specific product of the cells of one part, transported in the body fluid or the sap of an organism and producing a specific effect on the activity of cells remote from its source.
Immunity	State or power of resisting the development of a given disease.
Law of mass action	That the chemical action of a reacting substance is proportional at any moment to its active mass, which is usually considered as measured by the molecular concentration.
Metabolism	The sum of the processes concerned in the building up of protoplasm and its destruction incidental to life.
Me V	It is unit of energy commonly used in nuclear and particle physics, equal to the energy acquired by an electron in fall-ing and through a potential of 10^6 volts (million electron volt).
Molecule	The smallest particle of an element or compound that is capable of existing separately without loss of any original chemical properties.
Molecular Biology	That part of biology which attempts to interpret biological events in terms of physicochemical properties of molecules in cells.

Molecular field	A theory of ferromagnetism based on the hypothesis that below the curie point, a ferromagnetic substance is composed of small, spontaneously magnetized regions called domains and each domain is spontaneously magnetized because a strong molecular magnetic field tends to align the individual atomic magnetic moments within the domain
Molecular weight	The weight of any molecule being the sum of the weight of its atoms
Muon	Collective name for two semi stable elementary particles, with positive ' and negative charge.
Mounic atom	An atom in which an electron is replaced by a negatively charged muon orbiting close to or within the nucleus.
Mutation Nucleic acid	Alteration in form or qualities. DNA (deoxyribo nucleic acid) and RNA (ribo nucleic acid) built by four subunits named, adenine, cytosine, guanine and thymine.
Paroxysm	Sudden development of recurrence of symptoms of a disease.
Pathogens	An organism or virus causing disease
Pathology	The study of diseases, their essential nature, causes and development, and the structural and functional changes produced by them.
Pest	Any particular injurious or destructive insect.
Phenotypes	A type determined by the visible characters common to a group, as distinguished from their hereditary characters.
Polar molecule	A molecule having a permanent electric dipole moment, (electric

	dipole: a localized distribution of a positive and negative electricity without net charge, whose mean position of positive and negative charges do not coincide).
Polarity	Property of a physical system which has two points with different (usually opposite) characteristics, such as which has opposite charges or electric potentials or opposite magnetic poles
Polymer	Substance made of giant molecules formed by the union of simple molecules. For example polymerization of ethylene forms polythylene
Prodrome	Premonitory symptoms of a disease.
Quantum theory	The theory that the emission or absorption of energy by atoms or molecules is not continuous but occurs in discrete amounts, each amount being called a quantum
Quantum chemistry	Branch of physical chemistry concerned with the explanation of chemical phenomena by means of quantum mechanics.
Quantum mechanics	The modern theory of matter, of electro-magnetic radiation and of the interaction between matter and radiation. Differs from classical physics which it generalizes and supersedes mainly in the realm of atomic and sub-atomic phenomena.
Quantum electrodynamics	Die quantum theory of electro magnetic radiation, synthesizing the 'wave' and corpuscular' pictures and of the interaction of radiation with elastically charged matter, in particular with atoms and their constituent electrons.

Quark	One of the hypothetical basic particles, from which many of the elementary particles may in theory be built up.
Reticulo-endothelial	The macrophages system, comprising histocytes, monocytes, reticular cell etc.
Sine wave	A wave whose amplitude varies as the sine of a linear function of time
Soma	Whole of any organism except germ cells.
Stimulant	An agent which produces a temporary increase of vital activity in the organism or in any of its parts.
Therapeutic	Pertaining to the healing art, concerned with remedies for diseases.
Thermodynamic	Caused or operated by force due to the application of heat
Tissue culture	The science of making body tissue grow in culture medium outside of the body.
Toxin	A poison formed as a specific secretion product in the metabolism of a vegetable or animal organism.
Toxic	Pertaining to or caused by poison or toxin.
Toxicology	The science which treats of poisons, their effects, antidotes and recognition.
Virus	Smaller than microscopically visible bacteria, can be seen by electron microscope (size : 20 x 30 milli-micron).
Water culture	An experimental method of growing plants in distilled wa-ter, to which nutritive salts in certain definite proportions are added.

References

1. **Encyclopaedia Britannica** : Vol, 15, p. 185-205 (1959)
2. **David Bradney** : New Scientist, p. 404-406, Vol. 70, No. 1001 (1976)
3. **E.S. Anderson** : New Scientist, p. 194-196, Vol. 73, No. 1036 (1977)
4. **Roger Lewin** : New Scientist, p. 240-205, vol. 73, No. 1049 (1977)
5. **Donald Gould**: New Scientist, p. 689-691, vol. 70, No. 1006 (1976)
6. **Mike Muller** : New Scientist, p. 216-218 vol 70, No. 998 (1976)
7. **Heinz Henne** : Hahnemann A physician at the Dawn of a New Era, (Hippokrates verlag Stuttgart, 1977)
8. **Semuel Hahnemann** : Organon of Medicine, 1960, First Indian Edition, M. Bhattacharya & Co.,Calcutta.
9. **Samuel Hahnemann** : The chronic Diseases, 1976, Jain Publishing Co., New Delhi.
10. **D.S.Rawson** : The Hahnemannian Gleanings, p.538-543, vol. XLIII, No. 12, (1976)
11. **J. Boiron** : The Hahnemannian Gleanings, p. 451-462, vol. XLIII, No. 10 (1976)
12. **Lisa Wurmser** : Evolution of Research in Homoeopathy, p. 227-251, Souvenir, XXXII Interna-tional Homoeopathic Congress, (India) 1977.
13. **A.C.Dutta** : Homoeopathy, a Light Isotopic Treatment, 1991, p. 41- 52, B. Jain Publishers(P)Ltd., New Delhi-110 055.
14. **I .L.Finar** : Organic Chemistry, 1960, vol.1, p. 1-2, Longmans Green and Co. Ltd.

15. **J.M.Barry** : Molecular Biology - Genes and the Chemical Control of Living Cells,
(Prentice-Hall International Inc. London 1965).
16. **G.W.Roderick**: Man and Heredity, (MacMillan & Co. Ltd., London 1968).
17. **J.R. Oppenheimer** : The World of Atom, vol. 1, 1966, p. 462-500 (Basic Book Inc. Publishers, USA).
18 **J.R. Oppenheimer** : The World of Atom, vol. II, 1966, p. 1966, p. 1041-1525 (Basic Book Inc. Publishers, USA).
19. **W.F. Williams** : Encyclopedic Dictionary of Physics 1962, p. 594-595, vol. 5 (Pergamon Press Ltd., London).
20. **M. Lefort** : Nuclear Chemistry, 1968, p. 46-58 (D. Van Nostrand Co. Ltd., London).
21. **L.T.D. Vlasov** : 107 stories about chemistry, 1972, p. 210-212 (Mir Publishers, Moscow)
22. **M. Heissnisky** : Nuclear Chemistry and its Application, 1964, p. 33-34,
(Addision - Wesley Publish-ing Co. USA)
23. **Encyclopedia Britannica** : p. 169-170, vol. 8 (1959)
24. **J. Maddox** : Nature, 23 Feb. 1989, vol. 337,p. 685.
25 **J.M. Irvine, S.Riley** : Nature, vol. 339, p. 515, 15 June 1989, 'Scientific Corre-spondence',
(Department of Theoretical Physics, Schuster Laboratory, U.K.)
26. **P.S.H. Henry** : Encyclopedic Dictionary of Physics, p. 842, vol. 6
(Pergamon Press 1962)
27. **E.T.S. Walton** : Nobel Lectures, Physics 1942-62, p. 187-194
(Elsevier Publication)
28. **J.M. Tedder** : Basic Organic Chemistry, Part 2, p. 44-46,

John Wiley and Sons, 1967, London
29. M.L. Cohen : J. Science, vol. 198, No. 4318, Nov. 1977, p.713-717.
30. S. Berkman : Catalysis, Inorganic and Or-ganic, 1940, p. 33.
(Reinhold Publishing Corporation USA)
31. V. Singh : Science Today, March 1980, p. 43-51.
32. Encyclopedia Britannica : p. 923-924, vol. 22 (1959) p. 103-116, vol. 12 (1959)
33. Encyclopedia Britannica : p. 103-166, vol. 12(1959)
34. Encyclopedia Britannica : p. 892-911, vol 2 (1953)
35. Encyclopedias Britannica : p. 275-277, vol. 17 (1953)
36. J.A. Rabello : Science Today, 10,47 (1975)
37. J.K. Temin : Scientific American (1972), vol. 226, p. 25-33.
38. J.K. Pike : Scientific American, Vol. 225, p. 84-92 (1971)
39. M.H. Freedom : Nature, 255, 378-382 (1975)
40. Short Notes on: Chronic Disease and Theory of Miasm p. 15-58 (B. Jain Publishers (P) Ltd. New Delhi – 110058
41. Encyclopedias Britannica : p.43-48, vol. 23, 1959
42. J.T. Kent : Lectures on Homoeopathic Philosophy, First Indian Edi-tion, p.
85-170 (Economic Homoeo Stores Pvt. Ltd., Calcutta - 1961)
43. D.M. Kennedy : Transaction XXXII Interna-tional Homoeopathic Con-gress, p.
196-201, New Delhi - 1977.
44. D.M. Gibson : Elements of Homoeopathy, p. 18-29, M/s N.S. & Co, Delhi.
45. F- Bernoville : What we must not do in Homoeopathy, p. 12-56, B. Jain
Publishers, New Delhi, 1974

46. **P. Sankaran** : The Potency Problem, p. 1-30, The Homoeopathic Medical Publishers,
   Bombay, 1972
47. **J.N. Kanjilal** : What every Homoeopath Must know in order to Save Homoeopathy for
   the Man-kind p. 1-8, (Calcutta)
48. **J.H. Bon Hoa** : Journal of the HMAI, p. 37-40, vol. II, No. 2, Feb. 1978.
49. **H.J.Muller** : Nobel Lectures, Physiology and Medicine, 1942-1962, p. 155-157,
   Elsevier Publishing Company
50. **F.H.C. Crick** : Nobel Lectures, Physiology and Medicine, 1942-1962, p. 811-818,
   Elsevier Publishing Company.
51. **N.M. Teich et al** : Nature, 256, 551-555 (1975)
52. **H.M. Temin** : Scientific American, 226, p. 25-33 (1972)
53. **J. Cairns** : Nature, 255, p. 197-200 (1975)
54. **J.P. Hearn** : Nature, March 1976, vol. 260, p. 97-98
55. **A. Kessler &** : Nature, October 1974, vol.
   C.C. Standley 251, p. 577-579
56. **P. Paul** : J. Science Today, October 1976, vol. 11, p. 51-58
57. **F.S. Jaffe** : J. Scientific American, July 1973, vol. 229, p. 17-23
58. **G. Chedd** : J. New Scientist, Feb. 1976, vol. 69, p. 454-455
59. **G. Watts** : J. New Scientist, Feb. 1976, vol. 69, p. 452-453.
60. **N.M. Comber** : An Introduction to the Scientific Study of the Soil, p.3-14,
   (Edward Arnold & Co., London)
61. **L.J. Audus** : Plant Growth Substances, p. 5-11 & 116
   (Leonard Hill Books Ltd, London, 1959)
62. **H. Teuscher** : The Soil and its Fertility, p. 22-24
   (Reinhold Publishing Corporation, New York, 1960)
63. **P.P. Sinha** : Farmer and Parliament, May 1976,

vol. XI, No. 5, p. 11- 12
64. Emil Truog : Mineral Nutrition of Plants, p. 313-340
(Oxfold and IBH Publishing Co., Calcutta, 1967)
65. L.T. Evans : J. Nature, June 1976, vol. 261 p. 655-657.
66. Encyclopaedia : 1959, vol. 18, p. 30-38
Britannica
67. G.A. Stroble : J. Scientific American, 1975, vol. 232, No. 1, p. 81-88
68. Encyclopaedia : Vol. 11, p. 485-496 (1959)
Britannica
69. S.P. Chatterjee : Science Reporter, 1978, vol 15,No. 4, p. 260-63
70. A.F. Mascarenhas : J. Science Today. 19 76, vol. 10, No. 12, P.13-19.
71. S.N. Chakraborty : J. Science Today, 1976, vol. 10, No. 12, P. 19-21.
72. T.H. Morgan : Noble Lecures, Physiology or Medicine (1922-1941), p.313-328
(Elsevier Publishing Company)

Web Links to get more information about Positronium and Positronium complexes

1. Positronium- Wikipedia

2. https://aip.scitation.org/doi/10.1063/1.457116 (Formation and stability of a complex of Positronium with nitrobenzene from the study of the magnetic field effects.

3. The formation of Positronium in molecular substances (https://link.springer.com/article/10.1007/BF00929530).

4. Positronium in a liquid phase: Formation, bubble state and chemical reactions. (https://www.hindawi.com/journals/apc/2012/431962/)

5. Molecular Structure of Water-Like Positronium Complexes (http://przyrbwn.icm.edu.pl/APP/PDF/107/a107z416.pdf)

6. Electron-Positron annihilation (Wikipedia) https://en.wikipedia.org/wiki/Electron%E2%80%93positron_annihilation

Homoeopathy in the Light of Modern Science

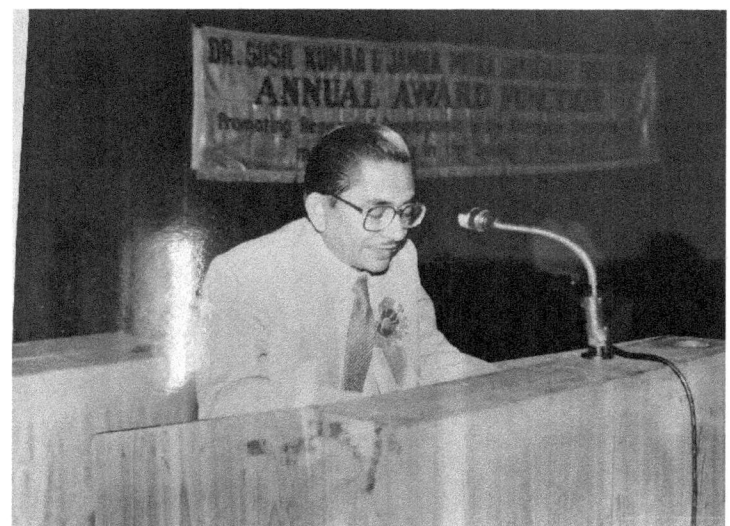

Dr A.C. Dutta delivering speech in the Mitra Award ceremony

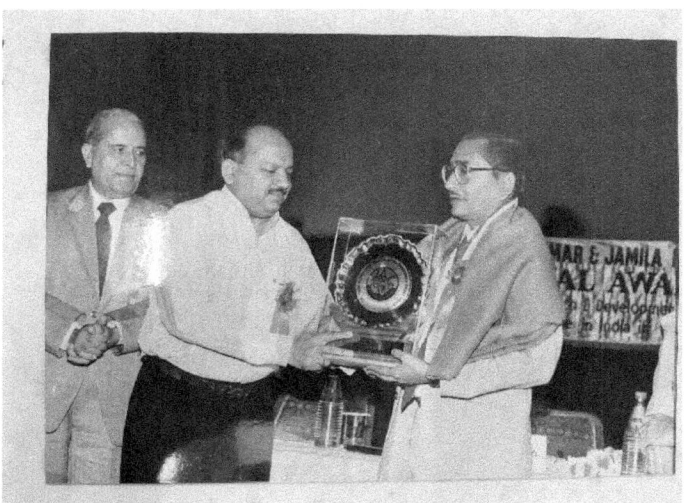

Dr A.C. Dutta receiving the Mitra award by the hands of Health Minister Dr Harshvardhan 1996

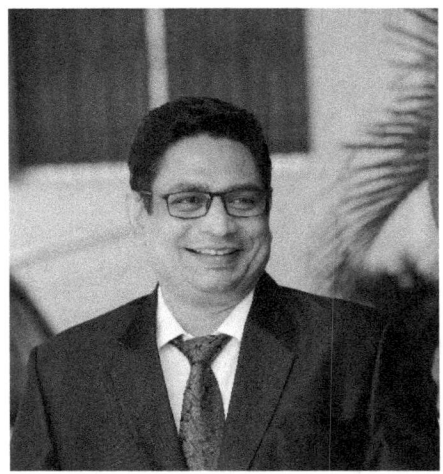

Would you like to conduct a Seminar/Webinar in your college/ Homoeopathic Organization ?

Drop a mail with your name, contact details and comments at drswarupdutta@gmail.com

We look forward to hearing from you.

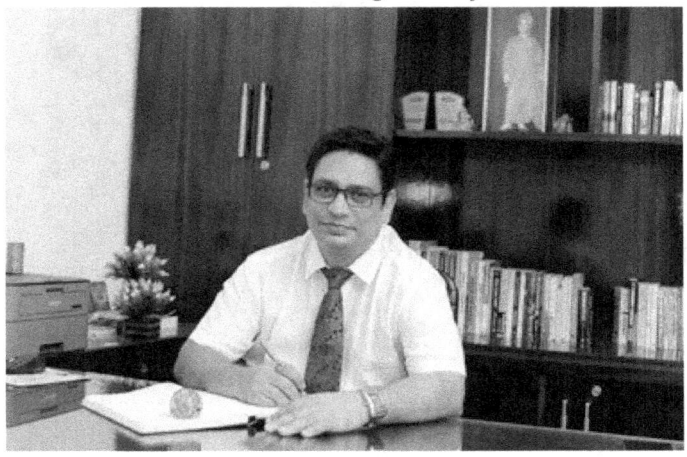

Homoeopathy in the Light of Modern Science